How Babies Sleep

The Gentle, Science-Based Method to Help Your Baby Sleep through the Night

SOFIA AXELROD, PhD

First published in 2020 by HEADLINE HOME
An imprint of HEADLINE PUBLISHING GROUP

1

Cataloguing in Publication Data is available from the British Library

ISBN 978 1 4722 7431 1

Interior design by Kyoko Watanabe
Illustrations by Danielle Ward

Printed and bound in the United Kingdom by
Clays Ltd., Elcograf S.p.A.

HEADLINE PUBLISHING GROUP
An Hachette UK Company
Carmelite House
50 Victoria Embankment
London
EC4Y 0DZ

www.headline.co.uk
www.hachette.co.uk

To all sleep-deprived parents

Contents

Introduction   xiii

The Science of Sleep   1

CHAPTER 1: The Circadian Clock   3

CHAPTER 2: Light Resets the Clock   10

CHAPTER 3: Sleep in Adults and Babies   24

CHAPTER 4: Broken and Immature Clocks   32

Step 1: Create the Ideal Light and Sleep Environment   41

CHAPTER 5: Using the Right Night-Light   43

CHAPTER 6: Day Mode and Night Mode   46

CHAPTER 7: Helping Baby Fall Asleep   54

Step 2: Create the Ideal Sleep and Nap Schedule   71

CHAPTER 8: Schedules   73

CHAPTER 9: Routines   89

CHAPTER 10: Naps   93

CHAPTER 11: Repetition and Flexibility   100

Step 3: Teach Your Baby to Sleep through the Night   105

CHAPTER 12: Signs of Readiness   107

CHAPTER 13: Gentle Sleep Training   110

CHAPTER 14: Is It Working?   118

CHAPTER 15: Sleep Regressions   123

CHAPTER 16: Sleep Increase   129

CHAPTER 17: Other Caregivers   133

CHAPTER 18: Understanding Mom—and Dad—Brain   136

Solving Common Sleep Problems   153

CHAPTER 19: Misconceptions about Baby Sleep   155

CHAPTER 20: Common Sleep Problems—and Their Solutions   159

Weekends, Vacations, and Time Zone Changes   165

CHAPTER 21: Weekends and Vacations   167

CHAPTER 22: Travel across Time Zones   170

Your How Babies Sleep Solution   187

How Babies Sleep Charts   191

Helpful Baby Items   193

References and Additional Reading   197

Acknowledgments   207

Index   209

How Babies Sleep

Introduction

As I watched my mentor, biologist Michael Young, accept his Nobel Prize for discovering the genes that guide our sleep behavior at the Royal Academy in Stockholm in 2017, I wondered whether my husband back in New York had remembered to turn on the red light when putting our daughter to sleep. Why? Because it's what Young, along with his colleagues Michael Rosbash and Jeff Hall, won the prize for that inspired me to try something new. His research in the Young Laboratory of Genetics at Rockefeller University in New York City—where I've worked as a postdoc and then a research associate since 2012—demonstrated that there are genes that regulate our wake and sleep cycles, and we can affect them in a simple way: by controlling our—and, by extension, our baby's—exposure to light.

You're probably wondering what this has to do with my husband and a red light in my daughter's nursery, so let me explain. You see, I'm a sleep scientist, but I'm also a mother of two. So I know first-hand the pain of sleep deprivation when your baby doesn't sleep through the night, and how exhausting it is to care for a newborn who wakes every few hours. We've all been there—it's 2 a.m., you're in deep sleep, and then you wake to the piercing sound of your baby crying out in what sounds like utmost despair. Dizzy and disoriented, you take a look at your clock and sigh at the ungodly hour, but you get up and stumble into the baby's room, trying to figure out why on earth she is so upset when she can't possibly be hungry again. I was that mom, too many times to count. I was living in this constant state of brain fog from chronic sleep deprivation, and it was terrible. In fact, I hated feeling like that so much that I used every brain cell I had to fix my baby's sleep. And it worked— because I used the science of sleep.

In our laboratory at Rockefeller University, we study the fundamentals of sleep. We explore why we sleep, how sleep is regulated, and even the consequences of sleep deprivation. Thanks to scientific advancements and research from our lab and other sleep experts worldwide, we now know a lot about the science of sleep. This book will give you a science-based program to help your baby get a full night's sleep and set the foundation for a lifetime of healthy sleep habits *naturally*, without resorting to typical "sleep training" methods that can be hard for new parents. Because this program is based on science, you will be working *with* your baby's natural desire to sleep, not against it. It will feel intuitive and gentle, instead of forced and challenging.

By using the method outlined in this book, you will be able to have your child sleeping through the night for at least seven hours by sixteen weeks of age. How do I know? Because I've tried it myself on my two children and with clients in my baby sleep coaching practice and have seen it work time and time again. When my first child, my daughter, Leah, was born, I was clueless about how to help her sleep through the night. But I naturally started incorporating aspects of our lab's research into Leah's bedtime routine, and used what I learned in the lab to minimize her night wakings and help her fall asleep more quickly after feedings. It worked amazingly well. As Leah grew and I had another child, I continued to refine my process and distill the insights from scientific research along with my personal observations into a simple method. Now,

> By using the method outlined in this book, you will be able to have your child sleeping through the night for at least seven hours by sixteen weeks of age.

two babies, five years, and many success stories later, I firmly believe that the science of sleep can help your baby sleep through the night more quickly and easily than you realize. I've translated the science of sleep into a program that works for real parents in the real world, and now I'm excited to share it with you.

Because this book is rooted in science, it gives you a unique edge in tackling your baby's sleep problems. What are those problems? Let's hear directly from the parents I coach:

> "It's been impossible to put him down for his nap."
> "She wakes up every hour at night and wants to be fed."
> "My three-year-old was a great sleeper from day one, but no such luck with the new baby! Help!"
> "I'm so tired I keep forgetting important things."
> "Putting him down is a daily struggle."

Does this sound familiar to you? Are those statements that you use to describe your baby's sleep? What about the following statements?

> "Today he woke up at 5 a.m."
> "I let her sleep in this morning."
> "He skipped his afternoon nap yesterday."
> "She went to bed an hour earlier last night."
> "I put him down whenever he's tired."
> "It's the weekend! Anything goes."
> "We're on vacation! Anything goes."
> "She's learning to walk, so she's sleeping worse."
> "All babies are different. My son is just a bad sleeper."

These kinds of statements and sleep issues are all too common—I hear them every day in my coaching practice. All of these problems indicate a lack of routines, a poorly established circadian rhythm, and a lack of understanding about the nature of sleep itself. Erratic sleep schedules that change from day to day are prevalent and take a big toll on the parents. This book will help you understand and fix all of these issues.

A New Solution, Rooted in Science

While there are myriad books, articles, and blogs about baby sleep, this book contains the sleep research and scientific knowledge to help you understand which factors affect baby sleep, and which don't. There's endless and often contradictory advice out there on how to "Make a baby sleep through the night," and "What's best for baby." While some experts advocate "baby-led" feeding and sleeping, others believe in strict routines. Cosleeping, baby-carrying, nursing, cry-it-out—these various methods are pushed by their proponents with almost religious belief, making a case for how vital these practices are for baby's health and well-being.

The reason parents are confused as to what to do is not a lack of information. The information is out there: on the internet, on the bookshelves, available for everybody to read. Many parents do just that. They read—a lot. I was one of these parents! The problem is that the information is not consistent and doesn't lead to a clear picture of what is the best way to get baby on a schedule or to sleep through the night. Every author of a baby book, blog, or magazine article presents his or her advice with conviction, but everybody has a different opinion. Parents end up trying different things, which don't necessarily work, and jump from one approach to the next because they are not particularly convinced about one method over another. That's because when it comes to baby sleep, scientific knowledge hasn't yet translated into common knowledge.

It's time that we brought our understanding of how babies sleep in line with the latest science. This isn't too different from the history of hygiene. For years, no one knew the true cause of many illnesses and diseases, because germs couldn't be seen by the naked eye. Just two hundred years ago, people still thought that washing oneself with water was bad, because water was considered toxic! But today, thanks to our advancements in science and technology, we know that germs make us sick. And we know that we can prevent illness by washing our hands regularly. Knowledge is power!

This book will arm you with the knowledge you need to help your baby sleep through the night. My program is grounded in biology and based on scientific discoveries from the past fifty years of research on circadian rhythms and sleep. My own work in Michael Young's lab gave me firsthand insight into the vast amount of data we have on the subject of sleep, which leaves no doubt about certain key aspects of sleep regulation. All we have to do is translate this data into our day-to-day lives. The best part: it's easy.

To succeed in your baby's sleep training, you are going to need two ingredients: the right method, and discipline. How do you know that my method is the one sleep method that will miraculously help you with baby's schedule and make him sleep easily and comfortably through the night? As opposed to other approaches, which might be grounded in people's personal opinions at worst and health considerations by pediatricians at best, my method is based on fundamental biological facts about our bodies and brains. Science has revealed important secrets about our inner workings, and some of them have been in place for millions of years of evolution. I'm simply taking the next step and applying those secrets to baby sleep.

> To succeed in your baby's sleep training, you are going to need two ingredients: the right method, and discipline.

To establish consistent sleep routines for baby, all we need to do is tap into that scientific knowledge. There are two main factors affecting sleep: the environmental conditions—specifically light—and our sleep behavior. The environment works in tandem with our behaviors to affect our sleep duration and quality. In addition to distilling the science into easy-to-follow advice, I will also help you maintain the number one most important tool for success in sleep training: discipline.

Once you understand the science and methodology behind this program, you will see why the How Babies Sleep method is the road to a peaceful night of sleep—for you and your baby.

What We Know About Sleep

Our laboratory studies circadian rhythms and sleep, and my mentor, Mike Young, won the 2017 Nobel Prize in Physiology or Medicine for his lifelong work on it. Thirty-five years ago, Young and his team of researchers discovered that there are genes regulating different aspects of circadian behavior in *Drosophila melanogaster*, the fruit fly, including the timing of sleep. Over the years, our lab's research contributed to painting a detailed picture of the molecular mechanisms governing our sleep behavior.

One of the most amazing revelations to come from this research was that the genes that regulate fruit flies' sleep are present in all animals—and even plants—on earth. In fact, these genes evolved to adapt to the planet's spin on its axis and revolutions around the sun. They are called clock genes and they function in most cells of our body. How do these body clocks know what time it is? A specialized part of our brain called the suprachiasmatic nucleus (SCN) is responsible for keeping time in our body and has therefore been dubbed the pacemaker or master clock. Clock genes in this master clock tell all cells of our body what time it is, regulating our physiology and behavior, including sleep.

> The genes that regulate fruit flies' sleep are present in all animals—and even plants—on earth.

What's particularly interesting when it comes to regulating sleep—both ours and our babies'—is the effect light has on the master clock. The master clock is synchronized to the light/dark cycle through specialized cells in our eyes, which transmit time-of-day information to the brain. The way this "entrainment" works is the same in babies, who are actually even more sensitive to light than adults. Therefore, a big part of my method is controlling baby's light exposure. In "The Science of Sleep," I go into much more detail about the various factors that affect our sleep, which form the backbone of this program.

The Importance of a Schedule

When my first baby was born, before I developed the program you're reading right now, I was overwhelmed by all the conflicting information out there. We had a nanny for Leah, a very sweet Russian lady named Nadia (name changed to protect privacy), who watched the baby while I went to work. Nadia started working for us when Leah was three months old. At the time, Leah's naps and bedtimes were still somewhat erratic, and I was hesitant to impose schedules on her. When Nadia told me that the most important thing for infants is having a schedule, I frowned. But now I know she was 100 percent right!

It doesn't always feel natural to mothers to impose a schedule on our babies. You might worry that waking your baby from a nap deprives her of sleep, or delaying feeding for a schedule deprives her of food. The reality is that sticking to a schedule from a few weeks of age not only is possible but will help baby—and you!—know what's going on, and what is going to happen next. It's important to stick to a set schedule, with regular nap, bed, and wake times. In this book, I explain why discipline is so crucial, and why repetition and routine are necessary for our goal: to make your baby sleep through the night. These same principles apply to adults, and by gently implementing the advice in this book, you will also vastly improve your own sleep and the sleep of everybody in your family. Moreover, your children will get a structured, calm, and well-rested start in life, which will carry on through later stages of childhood and into adulthood.

How to Use This Book

My goal with this book is to give you all the tools you need to help your baby sleep through the night by sixteen weeks of age. Much of my advice is very simple to follow, even if it's not commonly found in other books. For instance, adjusting the kind of light you use in the nursery and the timing of light exposure can make a radical difference in your baby's sleep. Here's what you'll find in this book.

> Adjusting the kind of light you use in the nursery and the timing of light exposure can make a radical difference in your baby's sleep.

The first three sections of this book form the foundation of my baby sleep philosophy. First, I explain the science of sleep, and provide a blueprint for the advice to come. My program will make immense sense once you understand why and how we sleep and what disrupts sleep. In step 1, I provide easy-to-follow guidelines to help optimize your nursery or baby's sleep space to create good sleep habits. In step 2, I explain how to create a schedule to reinforce these habits and help you and your baby establish a routine that optimizes sleep.

In step 3, I walk you through my very gentle and science-based method for sleep training. My goal as both a parent and a sleep consultant is to make this as painless for you and your baby as possible! So while I do encourage sleep training, I don't believe it's necessary to let your baby cry for an extended period of time. By this stage you will have made a lot of environmental and lifestyle changes to help your baby recognize when it is daytime and when it is nighttime. These changes will support the Gentle Sleep Training to make it as tear-free as possible while still being effective.

The last three sections help you personalize the program and troubleshoot problems. I unpack common issues like sleep regressions, how to adjust your schedule as your baby grows and needs less sleep over time, and how to prepare for travel and other events that can disrupt sleep, especially when you're crossing time zones. I'll also debunk common myths, like explaining why it's actually a good thing to wake a sleeping baby if her long naps are keeping her from a good night's sleep.

Throughout the book, I've dispersed How Babies Sleep success stories, stories from families that I've coached. These are actual accounts of different babies' sleep problems (with names changed to protect privacy), and I describe how we solved them using this method. I've included these to help encourage you along the way, and also to help you become your own baby-sleep sleuth. You can read those stories and test how much you've learned: Can you solve their sleep problems? Also, you can probably find your own baby's sleep troubles in some of the stories and learn what works—and what doesn't. Most importantly, you can see that we always apply the same three steps—create the ideal light and sleep environment, create the ideal schedule, and then conduct Gentle Sleep Training—for all babies, no matter what age and what the specific sleep problems are. My method is universal, and I want you to see that, because it will allow you to solve your baby's sleep problems today *and* in the future. I want to empower you to see the recurring patterns—and their solutions!—to take the right steps to better sleep yourself, and confidently know what to do.

By the time you finish this book, you will be a true expert in how babies sleep. Instead of making you follow strict rules, my goal is to give you the knowledge and tools that will let you confidently establish the best routine and habits for your baby and yourself. My guidelines are designed to get your baby sleeping through the night as quickly and easily as possible. But as you follow my advice, it's important to trust your intuition and know when to modify my guidelines to fit your baby's needs.

Trust Your Intuition

When I was pregnant with my first baby, I asked my sister, a mother of four, for advice. I expected her to recommend a particular book or childcare method. But instead she told me to follow my intuition. I didn't know what she meant at the time, but after the baby was born, I began to understand.

During pregnancy, we experience the effects of a hormonal cocktail, which lead to changes in brain connectivity and activity. What do these changes do? New moms—and dads!—experience the cries of their newborn baby in a much stronger way than women and men who have not just had a baby. An elegant study from New York University researchers in 2015 revealed how this works. Mouse pups, just like human babies, cry for their mother. Virgin mice ignore the pups' cries, while new mothers immediately retrieve the pups and start caring for them. It turns out that the "cuddle hormone" oxytocin is responsible for this behavior. New

> Both mothers' and fathers' brains are physically altered through pregnancy and childbirth.

parents—of mice or man—have high levels of this hormone. The study shows that it is specifically active in the auditory cortex of the brain, where it heightens responsiveness to pups' cries. Injecting oxytocin into the auditory cortex of virgin mice completely changes their behavior: They are no longer standoffish but exhibit the same caring reaction as actual moms. They go and help the pups.

I live in New York City, and because our apartment is noisy, I sleep with earplugs at night. When we had our first baby and moved her into her own room, which is separated from our bedroom by a hallway, I was unsure about sleeping with earplugs, because I was worried about not hearing her cry. It turned out that no matter how tired I am, no matter how deeply I sleep, the slightest cry is like a jolt through my brain and has me wide awake—despite the earplugs.

New moms report being much more sensitive to crying babies. I can attest to that. When I hear a crying baby—even if it's not my own—it is very hard for me to just ignore it. I distinctively remember a time when a crying baby was a nuisance and made me want to move away to avoid hearing the sound. Now it makes me want to help the baby!

While this heightened sensitivity might seem unsettling, it is actually an important tool to facilitate bonding between mother and baby. By experiencing baby's cries so strongly, you feel a lot of empathy for baby; you are extremely focused on helping him, and you pay careful attention to his needs. The increased sensitivity also makes you more observant. Your attention is directed toward the baby, and you watch him closely, trying to understand what he wants. Soon, you learn to read your baby's cues and know what he needs—even though he can't talk, or point, or control any of his movements yet. It becomes easier and easier to separate important from random signals, and your perception of your baby's state becomes better and better. There is a lot of trial and error that happens in the first days and weeks, but eventually what was first an active thought process—Is he hungry? Is he sleepy? Maybe he's cold!—turns into a deep understanding of that little person in front of you. Before too long, you will intuitively know what baby wants, at least most of the time.

I remember when Leah was only a month or two old. She was content in the baby swing in the living room, and suddenly she started crying. My mother was there, and she tried to play with

Leah to distract her—she thought the baby might be bored. I looked at Leah and realized instantly that she was tired. She was crying because she wanted to sleep. This was not a hunch; I was confident that she was tired and needed to sleep. It was not a thought process but an intuitive knowing. In fact, I almost felt like she was talking to me. Mind you, I wasn't hearing voices; I wasn't hallucinating. But the tone of her cry, her facial expression, her demeanor—everything spoke to me so clearly, as if she were saying: "Mommy, I'm sleepy. Bring me to bed."

When to Modify My Guidelines

Nature came up with an ingenious way to make sure we take care of our offspring, and your safest and easiest bet is to try to use the resources inside you that are unleashed by becoming a parent. What does that mean in terms of caring for a baby? It means that nobody will know your baby as well as you, and if you feel like the baby needs something, or something is wrong, then don't suppress that feeling, even if someone says otherwise.

> Nature came up with an ingenious way to make sure we take care of our offspring, and your safest and easiest bet is to try to use the resources inside you that are unleashed by becoming a parent.

Being a new parent is a constant negotiation of protecting and letting go, and nothing illustrates that better than the path to a baby who sleeps through the night. The guidelines in this book are designed to work with nature to facilitate your baby's natural sleep rhythm. But there might be many reasons why a baby can't sleep or is crying a lot that have nothing to do with sleep rhythms and absent routines. He might be too hot or cold, his clothes might be scratchy, he might be sick, or he might feel off because of vaccines. All of these things (and many more) can make the baby cry and prevent him from sleeping. As a new parent, you're naturally trying to spot anything that's disturbing your baby's well-being and eliminate those disturbances. Don't follow my guidelines if you feel like something is off, and if it makes you feel anxious or very worried.

I have kept these possibilities in mind in creating all of the guidelines in this book, and they can be modified accordingly. For example, if your baby is sick, she might need more comforting, more attention, and more nursing. It's also typical for a sick baby to need more sleep. She might want to sleep much more during the day and night as she fights an infection. If this is the case, instead of following my schedule to a T, you should allow your baby to nap longer, go to bed earlier, and sleep in longer—in other words, put my guidelines on hold for a temporary period. When, after a few days, she's back to her healthy, energetic self, return to her normal sleep schedule and get back to your routine. Most importantly, don't panic about sleep training during these times. Upending your baby's sleep schedule for a few days because of sickness will not affect her normal schedule, and she'll usually go straight back to her established routine as soon as she's healthy.

I'm grateful that you picked up this book and have trusted me with your baby's sleep. And now it's time to get started! I'm excited to share with you some of the fascinating research that has led to the How Babies Sleep method, so that you can get a better understanding of how this method works and why it's so effective.

A note to my readers: To simplify things, throughout this book I address moms instead of moms and dads. Please feel welcome if you are not a mother—this book is for everyone who takes care of or is interested in caring for babies and young children, no matter what gender, sexual orientation, or marital status.

INTRODUCTION
Key Points

★ Nobel Prize–winning research from our lab points to light as a major sleep regulator.

★ Understanding the science of sleep empowers parents.

★ Parents' brains are biologically altered to develop intuitive understanding of their babies' needs.

The Science of Sleep

In order to help your baby sleep through the night, it's important to understand what causes sleep in the first place—and what disrupts it. So in this first part, I will share what we know from scientific research about our daily rhythms and sleep, and how to apply this knowledge through specific, easy-to-follow rules that will improve your baby's sleep. After reading this part, you will understand why light has profound effects on our bodies, and that the timing and amount of sleep depend on very few factors, over which we have complete control.

To share this information, I will take you into the fascinating world of sleep research and show you how scientists worldwide tackle some of the most important questions of human biology. Our scientific excursion will lead us to research done many years ago in tiny insects, and as recently as last year in humans. After a crash course in hormone biology, you will know that we want baby's melatonin—a powerful sleep hormone—to be high at night and understand what it takes to achieve that.

Once you understand the science of sleep, we will apply all this knowledge to our day-to-day life with baby! You will learn how to use light to your advantage, and how to create schedules that make sense for your baby and for you. Step by step, we will translate general scientific knowledge into practical takeaways, and condense the broad research results into three specific areas of focus: light and sleep environment, naps and schedules, and sleeping through the night. You will learn how slight adjustments at home dramatically improve baby's sleep because they address the areas we know are crucial for better sleep.

But first, let's dive into what we know about sleep itself.

Chapter 1

The Circadian Clock

The day he learned he had won the Nobel Prize in Physiology or Medicine in 2017, Mike Young shared an interesting anecdote at an impromptu celebration at the Rockefeller University faculty club: The idea of a molecular clock timing our sleep and other behaviors was initially met with ridicule. "Genes regulating behavior? Nobody believed it." Yet, more than thirty-five years of research have revealed that our wake/sleep cycles (along with most other physiological functions and behaviors) are indeed regulated by this molecular clock that he and others first identified in fruit flies. This clock is the foundation of *How Babies Sleep*, and in this chapter, I will lay out the science behind it, including what the components of the clock are, where it is situated, and which factors affect it.

We each have an internal clock. This clock helps us organize our day by regulating our behavior and bodily functions, as shown in "The Circadian Clock" illustration on page 5. It tells us to go to sleep in the evening, and to get up in the morning. It tells us to eat breakfast, lunch, and dinner, and it prepares our bodies for absorbing and digesting food optimally at those times. It regulates our body temperature and our immune system. All facets of our mental state, including our mood, alertness, and drive, change throughout the day and are regulated by the internal circadian clock. What is the circadian clock, and how is it controlled?

According to this natural rhythm, there is not only a best time for sleep, at night, but also a best time for physical activity, in the afternoon, and a best time for bowel movements, in the morning. The scientific name for this daily rhythm is the circadian rhythm, from Latin *circa*, "about," and *diem*, "day." Together, this means "about a day," because that's the total duration of one of our cycles: about a day. Almost all physiological processes in our body are governed by a circadian rhythm.

All animals—and even plants—have a circadian clock, and it helps all life on earth to prepare for the sunlight and heat during the day and the darkness and cold at night. Plants need to orient their leaves so that they can start photosynthesis as soon as the first rays of light hit them. Predators use this clock to know when to hunt and where to find their prey; for example, if the gazelle is always at the river at dusk, the lion should be on his way to the water hole before then so as not to miss his prey. Animals in colder latitudes need to seek shelter before the sun sets to protect themselves from the cold at night. These are just a few examples from the animal kingdom illustrating the function of the circadian clock: to *anticipate* changes in our environment.

> Almost all physiological processes in our body are governed by a circadian rhythm.

What happens if you put a plant in a completely dark room, where the sun never shines? It will still turn its leaves toward its anticipated source of sunlight, and they will wander with the missing sun from one side of the room to the other over the course of the "day," and it will close its leaves to preserve humidity during the "night." All in complete darkness. The most astonishing thing is that the plant will continue to do that for as long as it lives. Which is not very long in complete darkness.

Interesting, you might say, but what does that have to do with me and my baby?

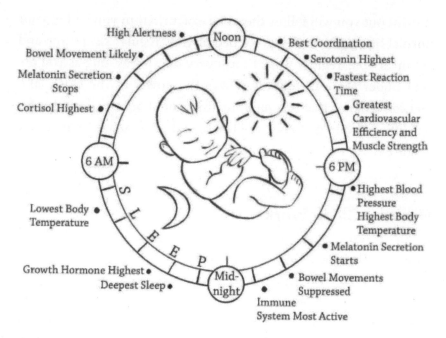

High Alertness •
Bowel Movement Likely •
Melatonin Secretion • Stops
Cortisol Highest •
Noon
• Best Coordination
• Serotonin Highest
• Fastest Reaction Time
• Greatest Cardiovascular Efficiency and Muscle Strength
6 AM
6 PM
Lowest Body • Temperature
• Highest Blood Pressure
Highest Body Temperature
• Melatonin Secretion Starts
Growth Hormone Highest •
Deepest Sleep •
Mid-night
• Bowel Movements Suppressed
Immune System Most Active

The Circadian Clock
Our inner clock creates daily rhythms in sleep, alertness, mood, digestion, heart rate, and a number of physiological parameters including the immune system and hormone secretion. Our clock makes sure that throughout the day we're optimally prepared for changes in our environment, such as being tired in the evening when it's time to sleep, and being hungry and ready to digest when it's time to eat.

The Power of the Clock

Say you normally go to bed at 11 p.m. and get up at 7 a.m. If I put you in a windowless apartment with no sunlight, no TV, no watches, no internet, and no other time cues, but with electrical light and food whenever you want, and books and as many movies as you like, and let you go about your day, deciding when you want to switch off the lights and go to bed, what do you think will happen?

Well, this experiment has actually been done, and repeated over and over again with various groups of people in different countries.

It turns out you will follow the same exact rhythm you had in your normal life. You will still go to bed at your regular sleep time and get up at your regular wake time, every day, for as long as you are kept under these conditions. That's the power of the clock, and you can see how that is something that would be very desirable for our little baby, to go to bed at 11 p.m. and to get up at 7 a.m. every single day.

How the Clock Works

How does the clock work, and how do we use that knowledge to get the baby to sleep through the night? Because of the earth's rotation around itself and the sun, which takes twenty-four hours, our internal clock has evolved to produce a circadian rhythm of approximately twenty-four hours. The length of one cycle is twenty-four hours, and this length is called a period. If the earth's rotation were slower, days would be longer and our periods would probably be more than twenty-four hours.

What drives our internal clock, and what tells us what time it is? Almost fifty years ago, scientists discovered that the clock is governed by a set of genes in our bodies, the so-called clock genes. Working at the California Institute of Technology in the early 1970s, the geneticists Ron Konopka and Seymour Benzer asked the following question: are there genes that are required for certain behaviors that normally happen only at certain times of the day? They were able to find an answer using the tiny fruit fly *Drosophila melanogaster* as a model system.

During normal development, fly eggs turn into larvae, which eat a lot and grow. Seven days later, during metamorphosis, each larva makes a little case for itself, called the pupal case. While in the pupal case, the larva transforms into an adult fly. The mature fly then breaks out of the case in a process called eclosion, ten days

The Cave and Bunker Experiments

The first researcher to test human behavior in the absence of society's twenty-four-hour activity cycle was Nathaniel Kleitman, who studied circadian rhythms in human subjects by housing them for a month in Kentucky's Mammoth Cave between June and July 1938. Here, he imposed an artificial regimen on his subjects: instead of twenty-four hours, day length was either twenty-one or twenty-eight hours. By monitoring their body temperature and heart rate, he was hoping to reveal whether humans would readily change their endogenous, which means originating from the body, rhythm to twenty-one or twenty-eight hours or stay locked into twenty-four hours.

He found that humans maintain their twenty-four-hour rhythm even when their external environment tells them otherwise—clear proof for the existence of an endogenous circadian rhythm.

German researchers working with Dr. Jürgen Aschoff conducted similar experiments in the 1960s, where they established a laboratory apartment in an underground World War II bunker in the Bavarian town of Andechs. Individuals were asked to turn lights on and off according to their liking and continue their normal day/night routines. Many student participants used their time in the bunker to cram for exams. By the early 1980s, when the program was stopped, more than three hundred volunteers had participated in the "bunker experiments." The conclusion was clear: even in the absence of light, humans maintain close to twenty-four-hour rhythms, providing further proof for an internal circadian clock.

after the egg was laid. Interestingly, eclosion usually only happens at a certain time of day—in the early morning—probably so that the newborn flies can spread their wings during the warm day and get accustomed to their new bodies while it's light and warm out.

To find out if there were genes required for the flies' regular morning eclosion time, Konopka and Benzer exposed the flies to a DNA-damaging chemical, or mutagen, thereby randomly perturbing the function of individual genes, and then watched to see if this genetic perturbation altered the timing of eclosion. Indeed, a certain mutation rendered the flies' eclosion arrhythmic: instead of all eclosing in the morning, mutant flies eclosed at random times of day and night. Furthermore, the researchers found two other mutations that, instead of rendering the flies arrhythmic, shortened or lengthened the flies' twenty-four-hour eclosion cycles to nineteen hours and twenty-eight hours, respectively.

In *Drosophila* research, there is a tradition of naming genes according to the problem they cause if missing. As the mutants Konopka and Benzer discovered cause alterations in the periodicity of behavior, the scientists named the arrhythmic mutant flies *period*, and the other two *period short* and *period long*, respectively. Years later my mentor, Michael Young, was the first to clone the *period* gene, thereby describing its genetic identity. It was this finding—cloning the first clock gene—that awarded him and two colleagues the Nobel Prize in Physiology or Medicine in 2017. The discovery of the *period* gene opened the door for understanding the genetic basis of circadian rhythms.

Building upon this groundbreaking work, our laboratory and many others have discovered a network of clock genes, which are responsible for keeping time in our bodies. Clock genes are expressed in most

> Our laboratory and many others have discovered a network of clock genes, which are responsible for keeping time in our bodies.

cells in our body. Each cell has its own clock. How are the clocks synchronized to one specific time? We have a structure in our brain called the suprachiasmatic nucleus, or SCN, which is considered to be the master clock in our body. The firing rate of the SCN neurons oscillates over day and night—it's highest during the day and lowest at night. The SCN firing rate instructs the rest of the brain and all our organs and tissues about what time it is.

Chapter 2

Light Resets the Clock

So if we all have clock genes and the SCN orchestrating our rhythms, how is this master clock reset? How does it know what time it is in the first place? The answer is complicated and depends on a number of factors we call zeitgebers (*Zeitgeber* means "time giver" in German)—but the main zeitgeber is light. When we get up in the morning and open the shades, specialized cells in the backs of our eyes, the intrinsically photosensitive retinal ganglion cells (ipRGCs), get activated by the light, and they transmit the light information to the master clock, the SCN. Interestingly, the ipRGCs are not required for vision. Indeed, blind people often show normal circadian rhythms because their ipRGCs still work, just not the rods and cones of the eyes, which are needed to see.

Once ipRGCs are activated, they transmit light information to the SCN, telling the master clock that the day has started. The clock is reset, and takes it from there for twenty-four hours. For people with a well "entrained" circadian clock, which are most people who go to bed and wake up at the same time every day, even if the alarm fails one morning and we don't open the shades at the same time, we will wake up at the usual time and be hungry, get up, make coffee, have breakfast, have a bowel movement, go to work, and so on.

Entrainment is the scientific term we use to describe the process of aligning the clock with a certain rhythm. To get the clock well entrained, we have to present it with zeitgebers. The main zeitgeber is light, but does any light reset the clock? The answer is no. Not all light is the same. Three aspects of the light you are exposed to are crucial for photoentrainment, or for setting the phase of your rhythm:

1. Time of day of light exposure
2. Light intensity
3. Light wavelength or color

Scientific Terminology

Circadian rhythm: The twenty-four-hour cycling of a behavioral or physiological parameter. Examples of behaviors that follow a circadian rhythm are sleep, activity, feeding, and bowel movements. Examples of physiological parameters that follow a circadian rhythm are body temperature, cortisol levels, blood pressure, melatonin levels, and testosterone levels.

Period: The duration of one cycle in the circadian rhythm. The human period is 24.2 hours on average, with small individual differences.

Zeitgeber: German for "time giver." An external cue that resets the period to a particular time. Light is the strongest zeitgeber; others include temperature and food.

Phase: The relationship of the period to real time or another oscillating parameter.

Phase shift: The adjustment of the phase to a different zeitgeber pattern, usually light. Flying across time zones causes a phase shift, during which the phase of an individual adjusts to local time. When this happens, we experience jet lag. Night workers are phase shifted to the normal light/dark cycle.

Entrainment: The process of aligning phase to a zeitgeber, usually light. During jet lag humans are entrained to a new phase. The body's phase is misaligned with the local phase until entrainment is complete. How long it takes to entrain to a different phase depends primarily on the intensity and timing of the light stimulus.

Amplitude: The strength of the circadian rhythm. A high amplitude is seen in people who go to bed and wake up at the same time every day, even without alarm clocks.

Intrinsically Photosensitive Retinal Ganglion Cells (ipRGCs): Specialized cells in the backs of our eyes that are activated by light and transmit light information to the SCN.

Suprachiasmatic nucleus (SCN): Part of the hypothalamus, an anatomical structure in the mammalian forebrain. The SCN receives light information from the ipRGCs, causing its cells to be activated and to transmit time-of-day information to the rest of the body, therefore also called master clock.

Light Intensity and Time of Day of Light Exposure

To test the effects of different light intensities on our circadian rhythm, Charles Czeisler and colleagues at Harvard Medical School attempted to shift the rhythms of human subjects by exposing them to light of different intensities and at different times of day. It turned out that shining bright light on subjects at the beginning of the night caused their entire rhythm to shift to a later phase, but light in the early morning caused the opposite: a shift to an earlier

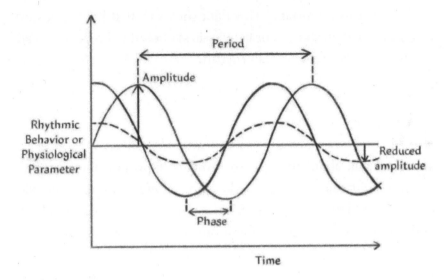

Circadian Rhythm Basics

Our sleep/wake cycle and many other behavioral and physiological parameters oscillate over day and night. The interval between peaks of a given parameter is called a period, which is usually twenty-four hours. The strength of the oscillation—how much the peaks vary from the troughs—is called amplitude, and the relationship between the timing of our inner clock to an external clock, such as real time or the time at a different time zone, is called a phase. Light exposure at unusual times, such as when we travel across time zones, causes phase shifts to our clock. Doing the same things every day increases the amplitude of the rhythm, but erratic schedules, as well as jet lag, shift work—or varying baby's bed, wake, and nap times—weaken the clock and reduce its amplitude.

phase. If a strong light was applied for three consecutive days either at the beginning or at the end of the night, huge phase shifts of up to twelve hours occurred, illustrating the enormous power of light. Such people were effectively shifted as if living in a time zone at the opposite side of the globe—solely by shining light on them. Even if humans were exposed to light only once at a time when they are normally surrounded by darkness, phase shifts occurred. Evening light exposure causes phase delays of up to three and a half hours, and morning light exposure advances up to two hours.

Why is this important? This data shows us that light exposure at a time when our body—or baby!—is supposed to be sleeping can wreak havoc on our circadian rhythm.

Light Color

Now let's talk about the third parameter important for a healthy rhythm: light color. Light is made up of different wavelengths that correspond to different colors. This is why prisms reveal a rainbow, and why you see a rainbow after a rain shower when it's sunny out. But most of us don't know that the spectral composition of daylight changes over the course of the day, as shown in the figure on page 15.

In the morning, the sunlight has a higher proportion of blue light, while in the evening the proportion of blue decreases and the amount of red rises, culminating in the sunset, which is almost devoid of blue light and bathes the world in pink, orange, and red hues. We now know that it is in fact the blue-enriched daylight that is responsible for most effects on the circadian system and sleep. When researchers used specific wavelengths instead of composite white light in their phase shift experiments, they found that blue light is the most potent in evoking phase shifts. In fact, blue light is sufficient to produce phase shifts of the same magnitude as white light, but green light, even though only slightly shifted from blue, is not as potent. Research shows that the longer the wavelength, the smaller the effect on sleep: two hours of bright orange light in the evening are much less disruptive to sleep than two hours of dim blue light at the same time.

Melatonin can go up only in the absence of light, and naturally rises in the evening after sundown.

Indeed, the photopigment in the ipRGCs, which senses the light and activates the SCN, thereby resetting the clock, is highly selective for blue light. Natural evening sunlight, which is more red and less

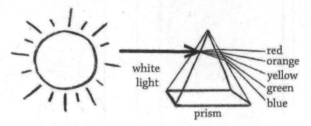

White light consists of different colors

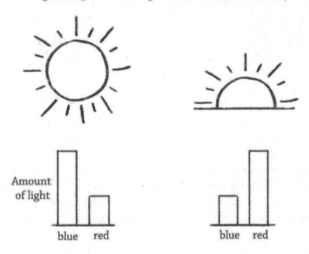

Light composition changes over the course of the day

White Light Consists of Different Colors

If daylight is shined through a prism, the spectral composition of light is revealed. Light consists of different wavelengths corresponding to different colors. During the day, sunlight has a high proportion of blue light, which decreases in the evening in favor of a higher proportion of red light.

blue, is not as potent in resetting the clock. How is the resetting effect of light mediated? It has been shown that SCN neuron firing directly affects an important hormone that regulates sleep: melatonin. Melatonin can go up only in the absence of light, and naturally rises in the evening after sundown, as shown in the "Blue Light Wakes Baby Up, and Red Light Encourages Sleep" illustration on page 16.

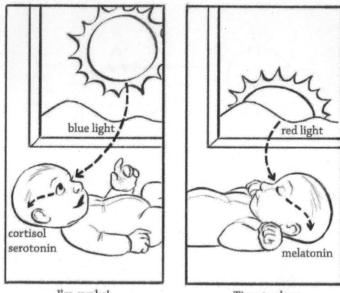

I'm awake!   Time to sleep.

Blue Light Wakes Baby Up, and Red Light Encourages Sleep
The high proportion of blue light in daylight prevents a baby from sleeping.
The blue light increases alertness by elevating the activating hormones cortisol
and serotonin and by suppressing the sleep hormone melatonin. In the evening,
light becomes less blue and more red, allowing melatonin to go up—and baby
can go to sleep. Avoid sunlight in the early morning, which will suppress sleep.

Artificial lights like incandescent bulbs, LEDs, TV, and tablet
and smartphone screens all emit blue light to varying degrees, signaling daytime to the internal clock and delaying the onset of sleep,
as well as reducing the quality of sleep throughout the night. The
effect of evening light exposure and specifically of screens has got-
ten increasing scientific and public attention in recent years. Many
scientific studies now show beyond doubt that screens, which are
enriched in blue light, significantly suppress melatonin and delay
sleep onset. In fact, in 2015, a meta-analysis of sixty-seven studies
aiming to test the effect of screens on children came to the conclusion that 90 percent of the studies found a correlation between
evening screen time and poor sleep.

Moreover, young children are especially sensitive to the sleep-disrupting effects of light. When Monique LeBourgeois and her colleagues from the University of Colorado Boulder exposed preschoolers to a "light table," at which they played for one hour during the evening, coloring on clear overhead sheets and playing with magnetic tiles to maximize light exposure, the results were staggering: the children's melatonin levels—which normally rose at this time of the evening to allow the children to go to sleep—were erased from their bodies by the bright light exposure, and remained low even after the light was turned off. The effect of light on the children was stronger than what had previously been reported for adults, leading the authors to hypothesize that young children are at particular risk for sleep loss when exposed to light at night. The reason for this susceptibility might be the fact that the lenses in their eyes, which transmit light from the outside to the backs of the eyes, are clearer than in adults, and become more cloudy with age.

> In 2015 a meta-analysis of sixty-seven studies aiming to test the effect of screens on children came to the conclusion that 90 percent of the studies found a correlation between evening screen time and poor sleep.

While there aren't yet any scientific studies showing that blue but not red light perturbs babies' sleep, I believe there is sufficient evidence to assume this is the case. More importantly, I have tested this idea extensively with my own children as well as with the many families I've coached and the results are clear: eliminating normal light at night helps babies sleep. These findings are crucial for How Babies Sleep and lead to a simple and effective rule: no blue—and therefore white—light at night.

Why We Underestimate the Power of Light

My home bathroom doesn't have windows. Instead, it has good strong lights above the bathroom mirror, totaling three hundred watts of white light. Such bathroom light is pretty typical, and is totally sufficient for, well, bathroom stuff: brushing teeth, washing your face, shaving, putting on makeup, and plucking eyebrows. Yet whenever I look into the mirror in our living room with tons of natural daylight, I am shocked at how many little eyebrow hairs I missed, and how many more, er, "details" there are in my face overall. My face in broad daylight: more pores, more lines, more wrinkles. More unevenness, more personality. Have you ever looked in the mirror in full daylight? It's truly surprising. Why is that? The answer to this question is directly tied to why the astonishing effects of light on our circadian rhythm and sleep are not widely known: because we don't really sense them.

Our perception crassly misrepresents light intensity. This misrepresentation helps us to seamlessly move between environments with vastly differing illuminations.

I once did a survey, asking my colleagues: What's brighter, office lighting or an overcast day outside? Living room lighting or sunlight in the early morning? The results were truly astonishing. We perceive light of different intensities as mostly similar; from the dimmest to the brightest possible light, from moonlight to bright sunshine, we perceive a fivefold difference at most, depending on the ambient light conditions. The real difference between these different lighting conditions is manifold, or many times, higher: your living room is actually ten times brighter than moonlight, office lighting is ten times brighter than your living room, an overcast day is five times brighter than office lighting—and full daylight is another six times brighter than an overcast day, making the difference between your living room and full daylight three-hundredfold, and not fivefold, as my colleagues were thinking. We simply do not feel how much more intense sunlight is compared to office light, and we can see pretty well in rather dark conditions too.

Wyszecki and Stiles describe in *Color Science* how researchers were able to exactly determine by how much we underestimate differences in light intensity. By presenting people with little patches of different light intensities, and also taking the light intensity of the surroundings into account, they concluded that we perceive

> We don't perceive the magnitude of light intensity changes across different light environments.

a thousandfold lightness increase, such as from moonlight to daylight, as only a tenfold brightness increase. Smaller differences, like the tenfold difference between your bathroom or kitchen lighting and an overcast day, are not noticeable for us at all.

This remarkable process is called adaptation, and it's a blessing that allows us to go back and forth between vastly different lighting environments. In this age of ubiquitous electric light, it's also a curse, because we don't perceive the magnitude of light intensity changes we encounter every day, and therefore we intuitively dismiss the idea that it's the light that's preventing us from sleeping. Our circadian system, however—our ipRGCs and the SCN—*do* perceive the light as it truly is, and have evolved for millions of years to respond to it in one way only: as a signal that it's daytime—and we should be awake. Moreover, the light sensitivity of the circadian system is extraordinary. Light as dim as candlelight, which has a low amount of blue light, is sufficient for entrainment, and light corresponding to ordinary living room lighting is sufficient for causing jet lag–type phase shifts. What does all of this mean for our babies? It's simple! We have to truly exclude any and all blue light during the time we want baby to sleep.

I know what you're thinking: *That would be all well and good, if my baby were sleeping through the night.* But how are we supposed to

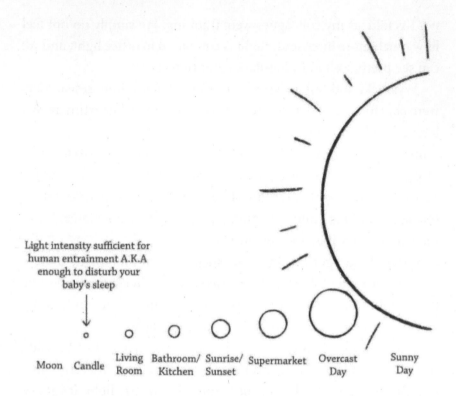

Light intensity sufficient for human entrainment A.K.A enough to disturb your baby's sleep

Moon Candle Living Room Bathroom/ Kitchen Sunrise/ Sunset Supermarket Overcast Day Sunny Day

Light Is Much More Intense—and Powerful—Than We Think
The circles illustrate the relative light intensity of the different sources of light. Our vision is highly adaptive to different lighting conditions, allowing us to seamlessly move from darker to brighter environments and back. Because of adaptation, we perceive dramatically different light environments as similarly lit. We might think sunlight is ten times brighter than living room light, but in reality, it's one thousand times brighter. We also underestimate the effect of light on our circadian system. Light as dim as candlelight is sufficient to shift our sleep/wake cycle; that's how sensitive our eyes and brain are to light. This means that you have to make your baby's bedroom pitch-black if you don't want the early morning sunlight—much brighter than a candle—to reset her clock.

nurse or feed baby, change baby, and placate baby at night if we can't turn on any light? There is an easy solution: use a red light, which doesn't affect ipRGCs, the SCN, melatonin levels—or sleep. Replace your regular light bulbs with red light bulbs to use during bedtime

HOW BABIES SLEEP SUCCESS STORY:
Light

A colleague of mine, Ellen, had a three-year-old, Dylan, who woke up at 5 a.m. every day. She told me that this was actually much better than before, when he got up at 4 a.m. My first question was: Do you have blackout shades? She said no, she only had light curtains. She had not considered the morning light in her son's bedroom as the cause for his early wakings, but I convinced her to give the blackout shades a try after laying out the scientific basis of my advice. After she got them, her son slept longer in the mornings, allowing his parents to catch up on much-needed sleep.

and for night wakings. (See "Helpful Baby Items" on page 193 for information on how to source red light.)

Now that we've figured out how to handle light during nighttime feedings, it's time to prevent the other very common issue with babies and sleep: waking too early. Just as you have to avoid blue and white light overnight, if you want your baby to sleep past dawn, you have to forget the idea that the "little" light that comes through the shades in the early morning will not affect babies' sleep. For one, that "little" light is forty to one hundred times brighter than your living room lighting, and one hundred to one thousand times more light

> Replace your regular light bulbs with red light bulbs to use during bedtime and for night wakings.

than required to reset the clock to a rhythm where the break of dawn is the start of the day. Do you want that? If not—if you want to sleep till 8 a.m. like me—get some good blackout shades. These don't have to be expensive: see "Helpful Baby Items" on page 193 for recommendations.

Food As a Time Cue

Light is the most powerful zeitgeber, but there are other zeitgebers that will affect the clock; in fact, almost everything that we do regularly might be viewed as a zeitgeber. If we eat every day at specific times, then those eating times will be zeitgebers and our body will expect food at those times. Just watch how your cats or dogs anticipate their meals: their bodies know when they're about to be fed! This will manifest itself as feeling hungry when lunchtime rolls around, but also as a number of physiological processes that occur in anticipation of food intake.

Indeed, researchers from the Department of Psychological and Brain Sciences at Indiana University found in 1995 that when rats, which are generally nocturnal, were given food in the middle of the day, when they were normally fast asleep, they started to develop what's called anticipatory behavior—they were expecting to be given food, so they woke up from their slumber and started to excitedly walk around. Humans, too, will change their metabolic rhythms if given food at a new time. British researchers found in 2017 that shifting meal times five hours later resulted in a shift in metabolism—to a later time.

Interestingly, unless experiments were conducted in constant darkness, behavior and sleepiness—and the molecular rhythms of the SCN neurons—stayed entrained to the light phase and did not shift to the later eating phase—in contrast to liver rhythms, which play a role in digestion and began to operate in a different time zone, causing asynchrony between the master clock in the brain and the peripheral clock of the digestive system. If the light/dark cycle remains the same, eating at a shifted phase causes a metabolic phase shift, but not a shift in sleep behavior.

Things get very different if there is no light. When rats were exposed to an altered feeding regimen in constant darkness, their whole rhythm shifted—including their sleep/wake cycles. This shows that food can act as a bona fide zeitgeber instructing all aspects of the circadian rhythm, but only if the omnipotent light is not there. Light is the most powerful zeitgeber.

So what happens when your feeding rhythm is well entrained? When it's time to eat, the stomach will produce acid, the gallbladder will produce bile, the liver will ramp up production of digestive enzymes, and the kidneys will get ready for salt excretion. All systems in your body will be ready for optimal digestion of your meal. With a well-entrained feeding rhythm, skipping meals feels especially disturbing, and eating at unusual times can interfere with concentration or sleep, or cause digestive disturbances, such as feeling bloated.

That is also why a feeding schedule is helpful for your baby, because instead of vague discontent resulting in constant crying and constant snacking, baby will be content and only hungry at eating times. Indeed, when the parents I coached were told to feed their babies at regular times instead of on demand, overall daytime fussing was reduced—and nighttime sleep was improved.

> When the parents I coached were told to feed their babies at regular times instead of on demand, overall daytime fussing was reduced—and nighttime sleep was improved.

Chapter 3

Sleep in Adults and Babies

When do we go to sleep, and what determines how long we sleep?

At first this may seem like a silly question. After all, we go to sleep when we are tired. But how is tiredness regulated? Scientists believe that our sleep timing is determined by two sources: one from the circadian clock, and one from a "sleep homeostat," a biological sensor that measures "sleep pressure," or how strongly we need sleep at a given time. As we have learned above, daily cycles of light and darkness affect our hormones and neurotransmitters, which in turn dictate rhythms of sleepiness and wakefulness. Cortisol promotes wakefulness during the day, and melatonin makes us tired in the evening.

> Cortisol promotes wakefulness during the day, and melatonin makes us tired in the evening.

These rhythms are the circadian component of sleep timing. However, sleep pressure is independently measured in our body, and also affects the timing of sleep. Anyone who has ever been deprived of sleep or had a disrupted night's sleep knows how powerful sleep pressure can be. Remember those all-nighters in college, cramming information into your brain for the test the next morning? Most likely, after the test, you crashed—and went to sleep. It was only past lunchtime, but you were exhausted from the night before and needed to catch up on sleep. Clearly your circadian rhythms of cortisol, serotonin, and melatonin were trying to tell you otherwise, that it was not time to go to bed yet, but your body said, "Sleep NOW." You passed out and, if left to your own devices, caught up on a significant amount of lost sleep, feeling better afterward. How do we explain this phenomenon?

Researchers proposed a model in which our body constantly measures sleep need—or sleep pressure—at any given time. Normally, our sleep pressure is highest at night, coinciding with our circadian rhythm. Sleep deprivation, however, doesn't allow our sleep pressure to go down to zero again through sleep, so we feel tired the next day irrespective of our circadian rhythm, because we have accumulated sleep debt. We go to sleep in the middle of the day, which is called rebound sleep; we're rebounding from a state of low sleep and high sleep pressure. Our body is working to erase our sleep pressure and sleep debt, even at odd times.

Rebound sleep is considered a hallmark of sleep. All animals that sleep will have rebound sleep after sleep deprivation. Even the fruit flies I work with will catch up on sleep the next morning if I don't let them sleep at night. How can I disturb fly sleep, you might ask? We have specialized shaking devices that give the flies a little nudge every few seconds, waking them up. Our exhausted flies go straight to sleep the next morning, even though this is usually a phase of activity for them.

To fall asleep easily, we need to make sure our circadian timing and sleep pressure coincide. We can achieve this if we go to bed when we're tired and sleep enough to be able to get up in the morning, but not so much that we are not tired the next night at the same time. We have a total daily sleep need that has to be

> To fall asleep easily, we need to make sure our circadian timing and sleep pressure coincide.

met by sleeping an optimal amount, enough to not become sleep deprived. In adults, this sleep need varies between people, but falls between five and ten hours of sleep, usually in a single block at night. The average person's sleep need is seven and a half hours in twenty-four hours.

Babies' total sleep need for every twenty-four-hour period is much higher. And their sleep needs change over time as they develop. I studied a meta-analysis of sleep data from tens of thousands of babies and children to figure out how much children sleep at certain ages and have displayed this data in the baby sleep chart on page 30. In the very early days, your baby sleeps most of the time—you've probably already noticed this! And as they get older, babies spend more time during a twenty-four-hour period awake and less asleep. The younger a baby is, the more quickly he gets tired again after sleeping—his sleep pressure rises much faster than that of older babies or adults. As he grows, sleep pressure accumulates more slowly: he will be awake longer after sleeping, and the intervals between naps will grow. It is important to understand that baby's twenty-four-hour sleep need is distributed across the day and night, divided into daytime naps and nighttime sleep. If your baby meets most of his twenty-four hours' sleep need during daytime naps, he will sleep less at night.

Napping

There's a common phrase used by parents and baby sleep experts: sleep begets sleep. And adequate napping is considered the holy grail of sleep training. But is that accurate?

Researchers from the University of Tokyo tested the age-old idea that babies need naps to sleep well at night. They tracked waking and sleep for a group of fifty healthy toddlers aged approximately one and a half years and discovered something surprising. Babies who slept less overall during the day went to bed earlier and slept longer at night. In contrast, babies who had longer naps, especially

HOW BABIES SLEEP SUCCESS STORY: Naps

Parents Claudia and Alex reached out to me to get help with their two-year-old, Liam. He is their third child, so Claudia thought she knew all the ins and outs of baby sleep, but Liam's reluctance to let go of night feeds caught her by surprise. Liam goes to sleep easily at 7 p.m. but wakes up multiple times every night, sometimes every hour. He goes to daycare and has one three-hour nap in the afternoon.

According to research (see page 29), two-year-olds sleep twelve hours in total every day. We just learned that we have a total daily sleep need, and if we cover some part of it during the day, we sleep less at night. Here we can see this scientific fact in action: Liam covers 3 hours of his 12 hours during the day, which leaves 12 − 3 = 9 hours for nighttime sleep. Currently Liam goes to sleep at 7 p.m. and gets up at 6 a.m., and those eleven hours include two hours of night wakings, which matches up perfectly with our sleep math.

So what to do? We need to cut the naps, and move bedtime later. If we want eleven hours of nighttime sleep and our preferred wake time is 7 a.m., then we need to put Liam down at 8 p.m., and reduce his daytime napping to the recommended one hour, as shown in the baby sleep chart on page 30.

if the last nap was in the afternoon, had trouble going to bed—and woke up more frequently during the night.

These results do away with the common but scientifically incorrect idea that babies need naps to sleep well at night. Babies need naps for an entirely different reason altogether: because their sleep pressure rises fast when they are awake, requiring them to sleep more frequently. Of course we need to facilitate naps, but the research from Japan shows an inconvenient truth: lengthening napping duration is directly linked to shortening nighttime sleep, and we therefore have to watch and gently limit those naps if we finally want baby to sleep through the night.

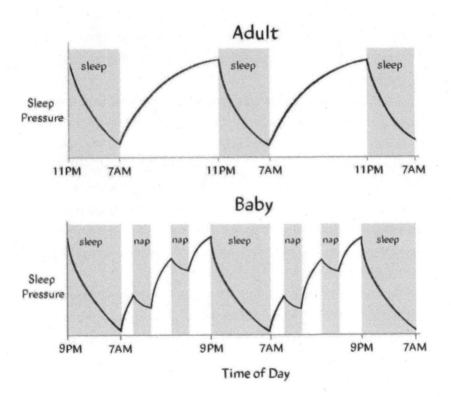

Sleep Pressure Makes Us Sleep
In both adults and babies, wakefulness during the day causes sleep pressure to rise, until we're so tired that we need to sleep. The only difference between babies and adults is that babies are more sensitive to sleep pressure, making them take naps, and they have a higher overall sleep need, requiring them to sleep more in every twenty-four-hour period. Too much napping reduces the sleep pressure in the evening too much, so that by bedtime, baby is not tired enough to fall asleep easily and sleep through the night. You need to monitor and limit naps to allow baby to sleep well at night.

How Much Sleep Does Baby Need?

Now that we know that too much napping is bad for nighttime sleep, how much sleep is necessary and healthy for baby? This is one of the top sources of confusion for parents, but fortunately science has a pretty clear answer.

While there are interindividual differences in babies' sleep need, overall their sleep patterns look and develop quite similarly. New-borns sleep all the time, yet two-year-olds only need twelve hours of sleep every day. Understanding how this huge reduction in sleep happens over time and how much your child is supposed to sleep during day and night at any given age is *crucial*, because it will help you adjust their schedule for optimal nighttime sleep.

Luckily, I did not have to go out and record tens of thousands of babies' sleep patterns to figure out how much babies sleep—other researchers have done that. In fact, baby sleep is such an important and accessible study object that there are now meta-analyses describing the combined findings of other studies. Barbara Galland and colleagues from New Zealand did just that in 2011—they surveyed thirty-four individual studies monitoring sleep patterns in various groups of children, from infants to twelve-year-olds. In total, the studies included 69,544 children from eighteen different countries. Using this huge data set, the researchers were able to determine global norms for sleep in children, showing how much children sleep on average when they are at a certain age. This data tells us how much children sleep in total during day and night, how many times they wake up at night, as well as how many naps they take and the duration of those naps. While the data shows that there are differences be-

All young children sleep a lot more than all older children, even if they started out with different amounts of daily sleep.

tween children and between countries, it also shows that there are global trends in sleep development. All young children sleep a lot more than all older children, even if they started out with different amounts of daily sleep.

We can use this data, shown in the baby sleep chart below, to figure out our baby's sleep needs at any given age: Are her sleep

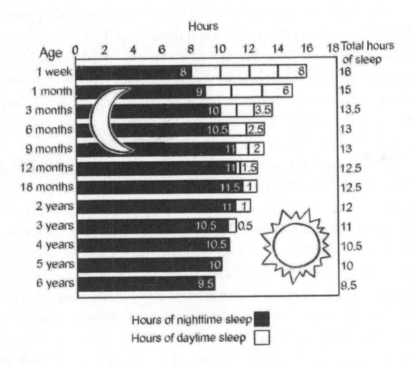

Baby Sleep Chart: Typical Hours of Nighttime and Daytime Sleep in Babies and Toddlers

This chart very clearly shows the typical hours children sleep during the night (in solid black) and during the day (in white). The vertical black bars in daytime sleep indicate the typical number of naps. To use this chart, find your child's age on the left and compare his total sleep with the number on the far right. If they are similar, look in the white bars to find the maximum duration of daytime sleep, and adjust baby's napping accordingly. If your baby already sleeps less overall, move on to the next older group—your baby is advanced and needs less sleep on average. Children around three years old often resist napping. When they nap, it should be no longer than one hour. But if your child doesn't want to nap, that's fine as well—it will eventually help with nighttime sleep.

patterns similar to the norm? If yes, great, but if she sleeps poorly at night and sleeps more during the day than average babies her age, we know that we're safe to shorten her naps at least to that average, knowing that tens of thousands of babies her age take shorter naps. Nap shortening is an easy and effective way to promote nighttime sleep, and knowing that baby's reduced daytime sleep is within the norm is useful information.

Chapter 4

Broken and Immature Clocks

Why are circadian clocks so important? What happens when they are not well entrained? Do babies have a circadian clock, and what can we do to optimally entrain it? Here are the real-world implications—and applications—of circadian rhythms.

Circadian Disruption

If we want to feel our best and optimize our activities during the day—including digestion, exercise, and even focus—it's essential to keep our clock and sleep pressure in sync. Yet many of us don't practice ideal sleep habits, and it's easy for our internal clock and sleep pressure to get desynchronized. We create a conflict between the circadian timing of sleep and sleep pressure by changing our bedtime, wake time, and total sleep time from day to day. This is a key point to understand when it comes to helping your baby and young child establish good sleep habits, so let me explain in more detail.

For instance, perhaps it's your bedtime, and your internal clock is telling you that it's time to sleep, but you're too engrossed in your book to put it down, so you read for another hour. You still get up with your alarm in the morning, but now you are missing one hour of sleep. You are more tired the following evening, and go to bed an hour early. You get extra sleep and feel great the next day, which happens to be Friday, so you go to bed extra late because you can sleep in.

This pattern probably doesn't sound so unusual to you. Many adults vary their bed, wake, and sleep times in this fashion. The problem is, it creates a constant conflict between our internal clock and our sleep behavior. The result is obvious: We are tired at many different times throughout the day, and our body is confused as to what is happening. Is it night? Is it breakfast time? Is it dinnertime? Is it bedtime?

Indeed, research supports that erratic bedtimes are strongly correlated with poor sleep. When 160 Taiwanese college students' sleep and wake cycles were monitored for two weeks, students who had regular sleep and wake times tended to report better sleep—but students who led a "student life" (just like your author in her college days), getting up and going to bed at varying times throughout the week, had more trouble falling and staying asleep.

Another variety of inconsistent wake and sleep times is *social jet lag*, which happens when you go to bed much later on the weekend than during the week and sleep in on Saturday and Sunday. Vast stretches of the population have self-imposed social jet lag, which dampens their rhythm and dysregulates sleep, mood, metabolism, and digestion—all those things your inner clock works so hard to optimize. On workdays, not only is their bedtime earlier, but their nightly time asleep is also shortened, creating a constant state of sleep deprivation.

> Vast stretches of the population have self-imposed social jet lag, which dampens their rhythm and dysregulates sleep, mood, metabolism, and digestion.

By sticking to specific bed and wake times—during the week, but also on weekends!—you align yourself with your circadian clock, which makes all your bodily functions, from digestion to sleep to mood, run smoothly. By living in alignment with the clock, you let the clock anticipate what you are going to do, and prepare your body for it.

People who regularly have to fly across time zones have a particularly hard time keeping a regular circadian rhythm because of frequent jet lag. By catching the red-eye from New York to Paris you lose a night of sleep, but that's not the main problem. You arrive six hours ahead of New York time, and the daylight signals to your clock that it is, in fact, not night but morning and a new day. Entrainment to a time zone doesn't happen overnight but takes a few days, depending on the new time zone and your light exposure. While the entrainment takes place over the next days, the external zeitgebers, including light and mealtimes, are causing a shift in the clock.

> By living in alignment with the clock, you let the clock anticipate what you are going to do, and prepare your body for it.

Experiments using twelve-hour shifts in light exposure and sleep timing showed that it takes three days for the endogenous, inner rhythm to adjust to the new time zone. During the time it will take you to fully switch to Paris time, you will experience the clash of your internal clock, still set on New York time, with the external, real Paris time. You will be tired in the morning, and wake up in the middle of the night, and feel hungry at erratic times.

Most people experience jet lag as miserable. That's because the shift doesn't happen in an orderly way; you don't just immediately phase shift to a new time zone. Research shows that phase shifts go through a phase of amplitude dampening, meaning your rhythm gets weaker before it readjusts. Our body is confused, stops preparing for mealtimes, and we have trouble digesting food, which is why many people report gastrointestinal symptoms during jet lag. We are tired because of the lack of sleep, yet we are not tired at the right time, because our body fails to produce melatonin, a sleep-inducing hormone, in the new evening, which is still daytime in New York.

The list goes on and on. People who are frequently exposed to jet lag are prone to develop a spectrum of health problems, including obesity and mood disorders that can be linked to a disturbed circadian rhythm. Shift workers face similar challenges as frequent flyers, and studies have shown that shift workers are more likely to develop sleep disorders, obesity, heart disease, diabetes, and depression.

People with certain kinds of sleep disorders, including delayed sleep phase disorder, have been shown to have mutations in specific clock genes, which affect the SCN firing, leading to an asynchrony between body time and real time. The result? Difficulty falling asleep, and a shifted rhythm that makes any kind of normal life hard to maintain. Getting up in the morning for work is a struggle for these people, because they can never go to sleep early enough to meet their sleep need. They live in a constant state of sleep deprivation, which has many adverse effects on their physical and mental health. In 2017 our laboratory discovered that one in a hundred people worldwide carry a mutation in a clock gene called *cryptochrome*, the functional analog of which was first discovered in our lab in fruit flies thirty years go. Our lab found these patients by searching for people who have trouble going to bed at night and waking up early—they suffer from delayed sleep onset disorder.

The Value of the Clock

The reason I'm going into detail about circadian rhythms and circadian rhythm disorders is to make a point about the value of entrainment, and about the beautiful function our clock has in making us healthier, happier people. By disturbing the clock, voluntarily or because of our work, we make it harder for the clock to run our body like a well-oiled machine, so to speak. Entrainment only works if two conditions are met: the zeitgeber has to be presented at the exact same time each day, and the zeitgeber has to be presented on consecutive days until the adjustment to a particular rhythm, called phase shift, is complete.

In our lab, we have different incubators for our fruit flies, with different light settings: we have one where it's light from 10 a.m. to 10 p.m., and another one where it's the opposite. We also have one where sunrise is at 4 p.m., and sunset at 4 a.m. We named those incubators according to cities in such time zones, so we have "New York," "Sydney," "Dubai," and so on. What happens when you move flies from "New York" to "Sydney"? Light at unusual times resets their clock, and they experience jet lag, but after three days their rhythm is completely shifted to Sydney time. The same is true for humans: entrainment to a twelve-hour phase shift of light takes around three days.

> The more consistent the timing is across days and the more often the zeitgeber is presented, the stronger the rhythm will be.

Conversely, the more consistent the timing is across days and the more often the zeitgeber is presented, the stronger the rhythm will be. Light pulses at night when it's normally dark have been shown to weaken human rhythms, as have gradual shifts in wake and bed times. The scientific name for rhythm strength is amplitude. Amplitude takes certain circadian behaviors or processes, such as sleep or melatonin levels, and measures how different that parameter is at different times of the day. A person with a strong rhythm will always sleep at 1 a.m., and never sleep at 10 a.m., while a person with a more variable rhythm will sleep one day at 1 a.m., but not on another, and might or might not be awake at 10 a.m. The first person has a higher rhythm amplitude than the second one.

We want a high amplitude in our rhythm, because that makes the rhythm robust to disturbances. If we forget to set an alarm we will still wake up, and at night we will still feel tired and go to sleep even in a strange hotel room on a noisy street. This plays out in the lab too. Even if we move our fruit flies to a special incubator where it's eternal night, they will keep getting up at the exact same time and going to sleep at the exact same time—even in the dark. Their inner clock keeps running with a high amplitude, even if external time cues are missing.

This is the ultimate goal when it comes to your baby's sleep. A baby with a high amplitude will still go to sleep at 9 p.m. and wake up at 8 a.m. every day, even at his grandmother's house, where she puts the baby down for the first time, and the crib is different, and the shades don't block the morning light as well. He will still sleep even after a very exciting day at the zoo, or after a boring day cooped up inside. His internal clock will make sure he sleeps.

Just like for adults, the alignment of sleep pressure and circadian timing is crucial for baby sleep. If your baby is tired at 6 p.m. one day and you put her down for a long nap even though she normally doesn't nap at that time, she won't be able to fall asleep easily at her bedtime, because her sleep pressure will be too low. She will still be tired, because her rhythm tells her it's time to sleep. But the discrepancy between sleep pressure and her internal rhythm will make it difficult for her to go to sleep. You probably know all too well what happens when your baby is tired but can't sleep . . . she will cry for a long time, and you will have to carry her around or console her in some other way before she can fall asleep. Consistency and repetition to bring sleep pressure and circadian rhythm into alignment is a key aspect of How Babies Sleep.

Everything we do either reinforces or disturbs the clock. The more processes we align, and the more behaviors we keep constant from day to day, the better

> The more processes we align, and the more behaviors we keep constant from day to day, the better our clock will prepare our body for whatever we throw at it.

our clock will prepare our body for whatever we throw at it. To put it another way, the clock is trying its hardest to set up and keep all physiological processes temporally aligned, with minimal energy expenditure and optimal function. The more we interfere with that temporal alignment—by having erratic bedtimes, by getting up at different times every day, by skipping breakfast, by eating lunch at noon one day and at 2 p.m. another, by having late-night dinners— the harder it becomes for the clock to help us prepare for the tasks at hand: sleeping, waking up, digesting, being alert, being tired, and so on. For adults, a weak clock can have detrimental effects on health and well-being, from difficulty sleeping and fatigue to moodiness, gastrointestinal issues, food cravings, and even more serious ill- nesses. Babies, who do not have good rhythms yet, are extra vul- nerable to erratic schedules, which will manifest in sleepless nights and lots of crying.

Baby's Clock

While we don't exactly know when circadian rhythms develop in utero, we know that they are formed by the third trimester. To understand how environmental conditions, specifically the main zeitgeber, light, affect babies' sleep and wake cycles, researchers from Yale University led by Scott Rivkees exposed preterm NICU babies either to constant dim light, or to scheduled light during the day and darkness at night.

When babies were exposed to light and dark cycles, they quickly developed a daily activity rhythm, with increased activity during the day and rest at night. This shows how important it is to control the light settings around baby—from birth. Other aspects of a new-born's clock are not mature yet. In adults, daily cortisol

> When babies were exposed to light and dark cycles, they quickly developed a daily activity rhythm, with increased activity during the day and rest at night.

rhythms normally peak after getting up in the morning, promoting alertness. In utero and in newborns, cortisol rhythms are flipped, with the highest levels detected in the late afternoon—when baby should be winding down. Melatonin rhythms are not even detected until two months of age. This means that newborn babies don't know what time of day it is; their behaviors and bodily functions are not lined up efficiently yet, and they are not aligned with the real time of day or their parents' preferred sleep and wake times.

In other words, when babies are born, their bodies are still disorganized; our job as parents is to help them organize their bodies in a way that makes life easier for them. How do we do this? We entrain them to a rhythm that helps them anticipate what is going to happen next. Babies are sometimes unhappy, and they don't understand why. By establishing a routine—with light, sleep, and feeding schedules—we help the baby learn that she's hungry or tired at certain times, instead of just feeling upset, and that her mom will feed her or put her to bed. This not only makes it easier for baby to fall asleep for naps and bedtime, but it also helps with an essential element of baby sleep—night wakings. Through entrainment, baby will learn that the darkness or red light is for sleeping, and naturally soothe herself and go back to sleep if she wakes up during the night.

The key to this is persistence. Over the next few parts, I will provide you with clear steps to create a routine for your baby and stick to it. Essentially, you're going to pay attention to your baby's cues, and then establish routines based on them. Once you have a routine, stick to it. Do the same things at the exact same time. Every. Single. Day. Try to develop routines for every single activity throughout the day: opening and closing the blinds, turning on red light (explained in the next part), feeding, naps, bedtime, wake time, play time, etc. The more things are regulated and predictable for the baby, the faster he learns which things happen at what times.

A regular routine will also help baby get better at those things— eating, sleeping, and so on—because she and her body will anticipate and prepare her for those actions and behaviors. It will also be easier for her to orient herself in a new place. When something different happens—for example, if you travel somewhere and she has to sleep in a different crib, or the food is different, or different people take care of her—the baby will adapt much more easily to these changes, because she will know what to expect.

Based on what you now know about our circadian rhythm, baby sleep needs, and sleep pressure, there are very clear and, thankfully, simple steps to take to help your baby sleep through the night:

- *Light:* No blue and white light exposure during the night and plenty of natural light during the day.
- *Schedule:* Repetition and consistency in feeding and sleeping is essential to entrain the clock.
- *Naps:* Baby needs to nap during the day, but avoid too much daytime sleep so he is tired enough to sleep at night.

How to implement these rules and to achieve our goal—a baby who has a consistent feeding and napping schedule and sleeps through the night—is explained in the following parts.

THE SCIENCE OF SLEEP
Key Points

★ Circadian rhythm and sleep are regulated by the molecular clock in our brain.

★ All light except red light resets the clock.

★ Repetition increases clock amplitude.

★ Daily sleep need is higher in babies and decreases rapidly as they grow.

Step 1: Create the Ideal Light and Sleep Environment

In the previous part, you learned about the science behind sleep and circadian clocks and how we can easily affect our sleep timing and quality by adjusting two things: light exposure and naps. Now let's put those scientific principles to work and develop the ground rules to help baby sleep. First up: light and sleep environment.

Chapter 5

Using the Right Night-Light

In the lab, I work with tiny fruit flies to uncover basic rules about sleep and rhythmic behaviors that ultimately apply to all animals, including humans. I've already mentioned how we have different incubators named according to the time zones of their light settings: in "Paris" the light turns on six hours later than in "New York," "Bangkok" is twelve hours ahead, and "Honolulu" is five hours behind "New York." Flies placed in a particular time zone rapidly adjust their activity and sleep patterns to the light phase, and within three days they are robustly entrained to the new time zone, even if it's New York to Bangkok. We can test the robustness of their rhythm by placing them into a completely dark incubator and monitoring their activity there. When we do so, the flies remain synchronized to the last time zone they were entrained to for the rest of their lives (fruit flies live up to four months with good care), even in the absence of light.

Because of the profound effect light has on the flies' rhythm, it is imperative to restrict the flies' exposure to light when they are "free-running," that is, in complete darkness. However, to be able to do experiments with the flies from the dark incubator, we have to be able to see them. Research in our field provided us with a trick that allows us to see in the dark without disturbing the flies' circadian rhythm: red light. We have red light bulbs and red flashlights that we use to handle the flies, give them fresh food, and perform our regular checks on them. The molecular clocks inside their bodies are blind to red light, allowing us to study them as if in complete darkness.

When my daughter, Leah, was born, I connected the dots. We know that our circadian clock, too, is insensitive to red light, but highly sensitive to the blue light that's a component of regular white light—including every light bulb you have in your home. I bought a red light bulb for the nursery, and used it exclusively during night feeds and diaper changes.

Just like my fruit flies, the baby almost immediately adapted

HOW BABIES SLEEP SUCCESS STORY:
Red Light

Mom Laura contacted me to get help with her baby boy Logan's sleep. Logan was full term and one month old, weighing almost eleven pounds. He was waking up many times during the night and Laura was at her wits' end. A few times he'd managed to sleep up to four hours in one stretch at night, but no more.

While Logan was too young for Gentle Sleep Training (introduced in chapter 13), establishing good light habits for baby from birth is powerful. Laura told me she'd tried blackout shades but hadn't used them consistently. I explained to her that consistency is key if we want to entrain her baby's clock to sleeping at nighttime. Laura started using the red light at bedtime and during the night and using blackout shades consistently, and reported that while Logan still woke up at night to feed, he fell back to sleep much more quickly—he seemed to sense that it was time to sleep. Teaching Logan to differentiate daytime and nighttime will help make sleep training more effective when he's old enough for it.

to this Night Mode and seemed to understand on a physiological level—facilitated by high melatonin concentrations due to the absence of blue light—that she is supposed to sleep at night. This part explains the most unique feature of How Babies Sleep: red light.

> Just like my fruit flies, the baby almost immediately adapted to this Night Mode.

So what's really so special about red light? Red light doesn't suppress melatonin and helps baby sleep, but is that all? When do we use red light? The answer is, at night, but is that enough for blissful sleep all night long? The short answer is: no, but almost. Proper light is the easiest feature to implement at home, even before the new baby arrives.

Chapter 6

Day Mode and Night Mode

Newborns wake every two to three hours to feed—there is no getting around frequently feeding a newborn to ensure weight gain, and to establish a good milk supply if you are nursing. But even newborns can benefit from an environment that helps them understand when it is day and when it is night, and to orient themselves according to the time of day.

I call the two settings Day Mode and Night Mode, and the goal is to maximize the differences between the modes so that baby's clock gets robustly entrained and baby sleeps at night and wakes during the day, with regular naps. Remember: Your baby is born with a master clock but without a clear sense of day and night. It's your job to help him figure out the difference, establishing lifelong healthy sleep habits. There are a few key aspects to the two modes, but by far the most important one is light.

Establishing Night Mode

When working with newborns and young babies, most parents are concerned about night waking and sleeping through the night. But once children grow to two, three, or four years old, the major complaint shifts to bedtime and early wakings. Many parents report that even their older kids wake up way too early and won't go back to sleep, and everybody in the family struggles with the mismatched rhythms between parents and kids. And too many accept the 5 a.m. family wake-up time as the norm. But you don't have to!

How do our bodies know when to get up in the morning? It's the blue fraction

> The goal is to maximize the differences between the modes so that baby's clock gets robustly entrained and baby sleeps at night and wakes during the day, with regular naps.

in the morning light that tells our internal clock that it's time to get up, as shown in the "Blue Light Wakes Baby Up, and Red Light Encourages Sleep" illustration on page 16. In the summer, this light can appear as early as 4 a.m. If there is morning light in the nursery at 4 a.m., the baby's clock will receive the signal that it's the start of the day, and the baby will be entrained to a wake-up time of 4 a.m.

How to avoid this? It's thankfully simple: Get blackout shades (see "Helpful Baby Items" on page 193) that will completely block out the light. Get them for baby's sleep area, whether it is a nursery or your bedroom, as well as for the diaper changing area, if that is in a different room. Make sure the shades are properly closed at night and try to minimize gaps between the shades as well as between the shades and the wall. Use tape if necessary to really seal the window and block all light out.

I've recently discovered a super-simple hack for installing these shades in five minutes: place adhesive hooks above the window and hang portable blackout shades with loops on them.

Check the efficiency of your shades in the morning, when actual daylight is coming in. Ideally, the amount of light in your room with the shades closed will resemble the amount at night. Why is this so important? Our eyes are supremely sensitive to light: we can detect light in the single photon range. While single photons are not enough to signal "It's morning, get up!" to the clock, very dim light

HOW BABIES SLEEP SUCCESS STORY:
Blackout Shades

My client Rachel, who lives on the thirty-sixth floor in a very bright apartment on the Upper East Side of New York, was agreeing with me in principle about installing shades in her super-bright bedroom to prevent her two-month-old baby, Lisa, from waking up at five o'clock every morning. But inertia and sleep deprivation prevented her from changing things—until I got her easy sticker hooks plus blackout shades. This quick fix turned her light-filled bedroom as black as night in the morning hours—allowing everybody to get their much-needed sleep.

and very short light exposure will trigger wakefulness, as shown in the illustrations on page 16 ("Blue Light Wakes Baby Up, and Red Light Encourages Sleep") and page 20 ("Light Is Much More Intense—and Powerful—Than We Think"). Therefore, make baby's bedroom as dark as possible. In the lab, we are extremely careful not to disrupt our circadian experiments by exposing the fruit flies to light. Still, accidents happen, and many an experiment needed to be repeated because an incubator door wasn't probably shut—a light pulse as short as five minutes is sufficient to reset the clock.

> By making baby's room dark, *you* will be telling baby's clock when it's time to get up, instead of the sun.

By making baby's room dark, *you* will be telling baby's clock when it's time to get up, instead of the sun. His room will be dark until it's wake-up time, and his internal clock will be entrained to a rhythm in which 4 a.m. is nighttime.

What about the evening—does bedtime also need a special light setting? You know the answer already. The blue light fraction in the

A Camping Experiment

Humans respond similarly to light as do fruit flies, as illustrated by a study in 2017 in which participants were sent camping for one weekend.

Before dividing the participants into two groups, the researchers measured the participants' melatonin levels and discovered something peculiar: melatonin levels were out of sync with sleep and wake times. Instead of peaking at bedtime and being lowest just before wake time, the sleep hormone was still high after subjects got up. Artificial light from light bulbs and screens in the evening was the likely culprit—as we know, the blue light that's found in most of our household lights (including screens) suppresses melatonin. The effects are dramatic: Many people report trouble getting up in the morning, being fatigued, and only properly "waking up" hours after getting up. At bedtime, many report trouble falling asleep.

In the experiment, one weekend of camping without any artificial light or screens eliminated the melatonin jet lag. Compared to the control group, which continued their lives as usual, participants in the camping group reported a lasting positive effect on their sleep, falling asleep more easily at night and waking up more alert in the morning. This study illustrates the power of sunlight.

When we are not camping, and when it's normal to stay up past sundown and want to sleep past sunrise, sunlight is detrimental to sleeping later in the morning, especially in the summer months, when the sun can rise many hours before your desired wake time, depending on latitude. (For detailed information about sunrise and day length: https://www.timeanddate.com/sun/usa/new-york).

In summary: increase light exposure during the day and reduce it in the evening and early morning to optimize sleep and wakefulness.

sunlight decreases in the evening, as illustrated on page 16. Melatonin production, which signals our body that it's bedtime, depends
on the light becoming less blue and more red. What does that mean
for our baby? Don't expose the baby to blue light in the evening. Use
a red light bulb in your lamp wherever your baby sleeps at night,
and where you will change his diaper and feed him. (See "Helpful
Baby Items" on page 193 for red light recommendations.) When
you put the baby down to sleep, turn only the red light on. This way,
in Night Mode, the baby's clock won't be reset to morning time and
melatonin production will not be suppressed—in other words, your
baby will sleep. The red light is not as bright as a normal bulb, but
it's bright enough to change and feed baby and orient yourself in the
nursery. When you get up during
the night because baby needs to
feed or is crying, turn only the red
lamp on.

> When you get up during the night because baby needs to feed or is crying, turn only the red lamp on.

If the baby wakes up in the
middle of the night or in the early
morning hours before your designated wake time and doesn't want to
go back to sleep, remember to stick to your routine. Keep everything
in Night Mode. Don't turn on white light, and stay in the nursery or
your bedroom with the red lamp on and the blackout shades shut.

Nursing the baby takes a lot of time in the beginning, and many
moms, including myself, use their cell phones to read or text to
pass the time. Cell phone screens emit light that contains much
more blue light than natural evening light, and it has been shown
that looking at screens, including cell phone and computer screens,
in the evening delays melatonin production and makes it harder
to go to sleep, as shown in the "Screens and Artificial Light Suppress Sleep" illustration on page 51. There is a simple remedy for
that. Turn on Night Shift (iOS) or Night-Light (Android) on your
phone or computer or install a free blue light filter program (see
"Helpful Baby Items" on page 193). It will prevent both you and

the baby from being exposed to blue light that keeps you awake, so that you can both go back to bed more easily after night feedings.

Eliminate all sources of light that are blue or green from the room baby sleeps in. The blue alarm clock and the charger with the green indicator light both have to go—use tape to cover them, if necessary. Err on the side of caution—the only light permitted in baby's bedroom and diaper changing area is red.

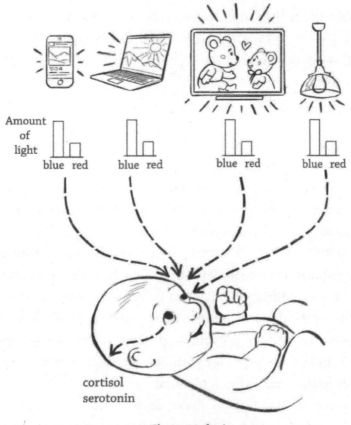

I'm awake!

Screens and Artificial Light Suppress Sleep

Screens and electric lighting have high proportions of blue light, which—just like daylight—increases alertness by raising cortisol and serotonin and suppresses sleep by inhibiting secretion of melatonin. Avoid exposing baby to screens and light at night, and turn on Night Mode on your phones and computers.

Establishing Day Mode

When it's time to get up, say at 7 or 8 a.m., depending on your personal preference and the schedule you will create in the next part, make a point of announcing the start of the day and implementing a routine. Say "Good morning," open the shades, and speak in your daytime voice when you get the baby in the morning. From now on, keep baby in the light until Night Mode, even during naps.

The goal is to clearly establish and differentiate Night Mode from Day Mode. Make a stark contrast between all daytime activities, naps, and feedings, and all nighttime activities, which should only be feeding, soothing, and diaper changing. During the day, don't be too quiet around your baby. Nurse and change her diapers in a bright spot, and in the beginning even naps shouldn't be in the complete dark, if possible.

> Make a stark contrast between all daytime activities, naps, and feedings, and all nighttime activities, which should only be feeding, soothing, and diaper changing.

Most newborns could care less about how light or dark it is when they take a nap during the day, but by exposing your baby to daylight during the day you are instructing her circadian clock that it is still daytime, and not yet time to produce melatonin and go into a longer nighttime sleep. Play with baby and talk to her during the day, play music, and go out and about.

In contrast, avoid all of these daytime activities, lights, and sounds during the night. At bedtime, when you prepare to put baby down for the night, start Night Mode. Don't let baby leave the nursery, don't speak louder than a whisper, and, very importantly, keep the lights off and only use a red light.

	Day	Night
Light		Red
Location		
Swaddling		
Interaction		
Noise		

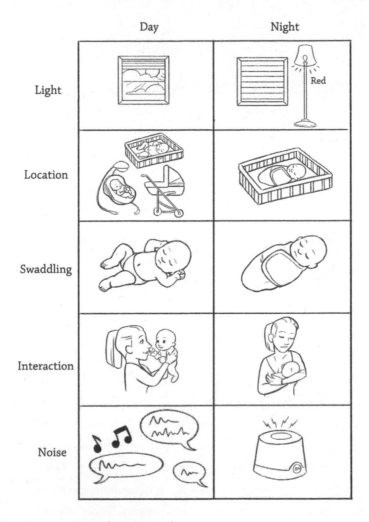

Sleep during Day and Night Mode

During Day Mode, make naps as different from Night Mode sleep as possible. Most importantly, don't make it too dark during the day. Don't make naps as comfortable for baby as night sleep, because we don't want him to nap endlessly. Don't swaddle baby for naps, and wake him up when nap time is over. You can use the swing for naps, but keep an eye on baby. You can go for a walk in the stroller to help him nap. During Night Mode, keep baby's room dark with blackout shades and only use red light. Always let baby sleep in his crib, and use swaddling and white noise to help him sleep. Minimize interaction with baby, only whisper if necessary, and place him back in the crib after feeding or diaper changes. Make it clear: night is for sleeping. Maintain Night Mode until it's *your* designated wake-up time, at which point you open the curtains and switch into Day Mode.

Chapter 7

Helping Baby Fall Asleep

Safe Sleep Habits

Approximately 3,500 infants die annually in the United States from sleep-related infant deaths, including sudden infant death syndrome (SIDS), ill-defined deaths, and accidental suffocation and strangulation in bed. After an initial decrease in the 1990s, the overall death rate attributable to sleep-related infant deaths has not declined in more recent years. Many of the modifiable and nonmodifiable risk factors for SIDS and other sleep-related infant deaths are strikingly similar. The American Academy of Pediatrics recommends a safe sleep environment that can reduce the risk of all sleep-related infant deaths. Recommendations for a safe sleep environment include supine (face up) positioning, the use of a firm sleep surface, room-sharing without bed-sharing, and the avoidance of soft bedding and overheating. Additional recommendations for SIDS reduction include the avoidance of exposure to smoke, alcohol, and illicit drugs; breastfeeding; routine immunization; and use of a pacifier.

Skin-to-skin care for newborn infants is recommended, but use of bedside and in-bed sleepers, sleeping on couches/armchairs and in sitting devices, and use of soft bedding after four months of age are to be avoided. The rationale for these recommendations is discussed in detail in the technical report at www.pediatrics.org/cgi/doi/10.1542/peds.2016-2940.

—Adapted from the American Academy of Pediatrics, "SIDS and Other Sleep-Related Infant Deaths: Updated 2016 Recommendations for a Safe Infant Sleeping Environment"

We all want baby to go to sleep easily and without crying, but infants and especially newborns need help going to sleep. Naturally, we want baby to nap during the day, but try to make daytime sleep less comfortable for baby than nighttime sleep, where you can and should try to create the coziest sleep environment possible. It's much easier to deal with a cranky baby during the day than to entertain a baby who's not tired enough at 3 a.m.! In addition, the more features of Day and Night Mode are consistently different, the stronger your baby's rhythm will be entrained. Think of sleep aids in terms of what we learned about the circadian clock in the previous part: Always using an electric swing for baby's nap at 10 a.m. becomes a zeitgeber for a half-hour morning nap, and always putting baby down in his crib wearing a sleep sack with only the red lamp on becomes a zeitgeber for his eight-hour-long nighttime sleep. How and where baby sleeps during the day versus during the night can help him learn that nighttime sleep is long, and naps are shorter. Step 2 will provide more detailed information about how to develop a schedule and determine the ideal times to put baby down for bed and wake him up.

How and where baby sleeps during the day versus during the night can help him learn that nighttime sleep is long, and naps are shorter.

Learning to Self-Soothe

How Babies Sleep will lead to established sleep times that allow baby to fall asleep quickly. Still, there will be many times, especially in the first few months, when putting her down will be challenging. The goal is for her to learn to self-soothe, so try not to pick baby up but leave her in her crib, swing, or stroller while soothing her. *Self-soothing* is the most important skill baby needs to acquire to sleep through the night, and it is wise to start encouraging it from the start. Picking baby up and carrying her around should only be used as the last resort to calm her down.

The concept of self-soothing as an essential part of sleep training dates back to Dr. Richard Ferber, who developed a model in his popular book *Solve Your Child's Sleep Problems* describing how parents interfere with baby's night sleep by forming inadvertent sleep associations. Parents often respond very quickly to babies' night wakings, take babies out of their cribs, hold them, and feed them to get them back to sleep. Ferber suggests that these behaviors promote specific sleep associations in babies. Babies learn to expect these parental interventions to go to sleep, and fail to learn to self-soothe. The result? Baby keeps waking up at night and cries for his parents, and nobody sleeps.

Ferber's method of sleep training, which involves letting a baby cry at night without being picked up for gradually increasing periods of time until the baby learns to self-soothe, became so popular that it's often referred to as Ferberizing. In fact, you've probably heard of this method or heard other parents talk about the "cry it out" method.

Ferber's model was put to the test when pediatricians from the Boston City Hospital informed one group of parents about self-soothing at their babies' four-month checkup, and compared night sleep in this group to an uninformed one at the babies' nine-month checkup. As hypothesized, teaching baby to self-soothe resulted in a 50 percent decrease in frequent night wakings in the informed group. We can also understand Ferber's insights from a circadian entrainment perspective: Consistently responding to baby's cues in the middle of the night entrains baby to await parental intervention rather than going back to sleep by herself.

While Ferber's method may be effective, it's also criticized for being challenging for parents to do, which is why I propose a more baby- and parent-friendly Gentle Sleep Training method, which I share in chapter 13.

How can we aid baby in falling asleep? Here are some common and useful techniques to calm baby and encourage rest:

- Swaddling
- Rocking
- Shushing
- Singing
- White noise
- Electric swing
- Fresh air (opening the window or going outside)
- Going for a walk in the stroller
- Going for a walk wearing baby in a carrier
- Nursing/feeding (see "human pacifier" in chapter 8)
- Pacifier (not recommended, see below)
- Muslin blanket to suckle on (better than pacifier)
- Carrying around
- Stuffed animal (for older baby or toddler)
- Blanket (for older baby or toddler)

You can use some of these techniques to help baby calm down when he is crying and to help him fall asleep. Remember, it is crucial baby doesn't sleep all day (see chapter 10), so use these methods sparingly during the day. For example, you can use the electric swing to help baby fall asleep, but don't keep it on for hours so he sleeps all day. Turn it off when nap time is over, so he wakes up naturally.

Below is a more detailed discussion of how to use some of the sleep aids in a way that helps baby nap, but also promotes our ultimate goal: getting baby to sleep through the night.

Swaddling

Swaddling a newborn can be extremely useful to help her go to sleep, because she is used to the cozy tightness in the womb, where her arm and leg movements were restricted. Newborns have a falling reflex called Moro reflex, where the baby instinctively throws up her arms when she feels like she's falling, in order to protect herself. This reflex slowly disappears by the age of four to six months. While babies sleep, normally occurring twitching motions trigger this reflex and then their flailing arms startle them awake. This makes it harder for baby to go to sleep and stay asleep, and restricting arm movement helps with that. Swaddles re-create that comforting tightness of the womb and prevent arousal from the Moro reflex, and many mothers—myself included—can attest to the power of swaddles.

Their effectiveness isn't just anecdotal; it has been tested in a sleep laboratory at Washington University in St. Louis. Using a variety of measures, including polysomnography to detect electrical activity in the brain to record sleep, electromyograms for muscle activity, and specialized swaddles that detect babies' movements, the researchers were able to prove that swaddling reduces startles and arousals during sleep by up to 90 percent compared to unswaddled babies.

While swaddles seem the perfect way to promote baby sleep, it is key to use swaddling only during the night, otherwise your baby will sleep too much during the day, which will disrupt nighttime sleep. Use other techniques to help baby sleep during the day (like swings, walking in the stroller, fresh air) and reserve this ultimate sleep tool for when you really need it—at night. You can use swaddles until baby learns to roll over, which usually happens around five to six months, but can happen earlier. At that time, it's not safe to swaddle anymore, because baby might roll over on his tummy, but can't use his arms to adjust his position. He might lie on his face and it could be hard for him to breathe that way. Once you've seen baby roll over even once in either direction, stop swaddling.

It's scary to stop using this helpful sleep tool from one night to the next. Instead of a swaddle, introduce a sleep sack, which is a wearable blanket that allows baby to move his arms freely. Fortunately, baby's sleep won't suffer after switching from swaddle to sleep sack, if all other Night Mode factors are still in place. That's the advantage of How Babies Sleep: You will have entrained baby to a strong rhythm using a multitude of cues including light, schedules, and routines. Swaddling was only a small part of it. Stopping swaddling while still having the same bedtime routine and making sure baby is tired at night will result in a baby that happily sleeps even when his arms are suddenly not constrained anymore.

Eye Contact

Avoid eye contact when putting a baby down. It is a longstanding notion in psychology research—and familiar to every one of us—that being looked at increases our arousal and alters our brain patterns. Locking eyes with mom is so exciting for baby that she becomes more alert. That's the opposite of what she needs when it's time to sleep. So make a point of directing your gaze onto her chin or belly so that she can calm down more easily.

Create a Designated Space for Night Sleep

If possible, it is a great idea to have baby nap in a different spot than where he sleeps at night. At night, always put him in his crib, which will always be in the same spot. For naps, use a different crib or bassinet, or let him sleep in a baby swing or while out for a walk in the stroller during the day—any of these are great options.

HOW BABIES SLEEP SUCCESS STORY:
Sleeping in the Stroller

One of my favorite stories is helping Max, a new father who complained about nap time. As Max explained to me, his baby, Olympia, had the hardest time falling asleep for her afternoon nap unless being bounced in a carrier. It was summertime and the weather was nice, so I suggested he go for a walk with Olympia instead, every day at the same time, to help her fall asleep—and help him get out of the house, a routine that provides much-needed change from staying inside. A week later, Max reported that Olympia had been sleeping like a rock during her afternoon nap in the stroller, and that he and his wife had been enjoying their afternoon break walking around the neighborhood. It was a win-win.

White Noise

Many parents swear by white noise as a baby sleep tool. In 1990 scientists in London reported that white noise allows 80 percent of two- to seven-day-old newborns to fall asleep within five minutes, while only 20 percent of a control group without white noise fell asleep in that time. White noise drowns out any ambient sounds that might disturb baby's sleep, but there is also a soothing quality to the noise itself. It's thought that white noise mimics the sounds the baby is exposed to while in the womb.

While white noise is a great sleep tool, use it sparingly, as its effect wears off. Turn it off during night feedings so you can use it again if your baby starts crying when you put him back down. Don't use white noise during the day for naps. If it is used only at night, it will become another signal for baby that it's nighttime, and time for night sleep. During the day, you can use different sounds to help baby sleep. Many baby swings have sounds built in, like lullaby music or nature sounds, and using them to soothe baby works for many parents. There are a variety of white noise machines and smartphone apps available (see "Helpful Baby Items" on page 193).

Pacifiers

When your baby is crying, you are willing to do almost anything to make her stop. I never liked the idea of using a pacifier, yet I tried to give them to both Leah and Noah out of desperation. Leah made it easy: she spit the pacifier right out and that was the end of it. Noah, on the other hand, took it, and what a peaceful first month we had. If I had just fed him and he was fussy—pacifier. Baby was happy and content, and the pacifier helped him fall asleep. We barely heard him cry during the day.

At night it was a different story. He woke up many times during the night and started crying, and I needed to either feed him or give him the pacifier to soothe him. Around week five it dawned on me: I had effectively trained Noah to need the pacifier to fall asleep. During the day that is no big deal; you just pop it right back in once it falls out. At night it means you will wake up many times to put the pacifier back in baby's mouth when he cries, because he cannot fall asleep without it. My baby was addicted to the pacifier!

I realized the pacifier was prolonging his path to self-soothing, so I made a radical decision. Cold turkey pacifier detox. One day we threw out all pacifiers and started the reprogramming. For about twenty-four hours we had a very cranky baby on our hands, and I won't deny I eventually broke down and abandoned my feeding schedule to nurse him whenever he got upset. For a while I turned into a human pacifier. Gradually, I reduced nursing as a soothing agent until Noah was back on his schedule.

While many parents swear by pacifiers and they might reduce the risk of SIDS (sudden infant death syndrome, an unexplained death of babies less than one year old, which usually occurs during sleep and has been linked to unsafe crib bedding), according to the American Academy of Pediatrics, I cannot recommend them based on my personal experience and also from working with other parents who have experienced similar problems. A less addictive oral soothing alternative is a muslin blanket. Starting around four months, Noah loved to hold the fabric in his hands and sometimes suckle on it a little bit. The lightweight, transparent muslin fabric is breathable, so you don't have to worry about SIDS. Still, use the muslin only for daytime naps, and keep an eye on baby when you do.

Where Should Your Baby Sleep?

Whether to sleep with your baby in your bed or in your room as opposed to in a crib in a separate room is a widely contested point in the parenting community. "Infant-cued" parenting involves bed-sharing and avoiding any crying. While it is very distressing for parents to hear their baby cry, is this the best way to help baby sleep through the night?

Apart from safety considerations—the AAP opposes bed-sharing due to an increased risk of SIDS—there is good evidence that creating space for baby to learn how to self-soothe strongly helps with sleeping through the night. In 2017 researchers from University College London compared infants who coslept with their parents to babies who had their own crib, using video analysis and sleep diaries. They found that parents who cosleep with babies in their bed respond to night wakings within seconds and feed immediately. Parents whose babies sleep in a crib respond to their baby's waking slightly slower, and also delay feeding baby compared to bed-sharing babies. Now here is the twist: The scientists found that at three months of age, only 25 percent of babies from the bed-sharing group slept more than five hours at night. In contrast, 72 percent of babies from the crib group, where parents had consistently waited for at least one minute to soothe and feed baby, were sleeping more than five hours at night. In other words, delaying feeding a young baby *by as little as one minute* has profound effects on how quickly baby sleeps through the night. Delaying soothing and feeding when baby is right there next to you is nearly impossible, but having baby in her own crib, or, even better, in her own room, allows parents to be disciplined and thereby teach baby to self-soothe.

What about having baby in his crib in your room versus his own room? While it makes sense to have him in your room in the first few weeks while he is feeding all the time—having him close by will minimize your sleep disruptions—after a certain point it makes sense to put him in his own room, if this is an option. You will notice that he is highly sensitive to sounds in the bedroom, and mom's turning in bed or daddy's snoring will often wake baby. Conversely, baby's manifold and varied noises and grunts, while adorable, can be disruptive to your sleep.

Indeed, a 2015 study conducted by scientists in Israel showed just that: Letting baby sleep in her own room significantly improved both infants' and mothers' sleep. The researchers compared sleep in infants and mothers who coslept with baby in the parents' room to that of babies in their own room and found that mothers who coslept reported more night wakings and poorer sleep at three and six months of age compared to mothers whose infants slept in their own room. In other words, putting baby in her room (either within earshot or with a baby monitor so that you can hear when she wakes) will at the very least improve *your* sleep, and often also your baby's. When you will start trying to extend baby's nighttime sleep phases, not having her in your room will be much easier, because it will allow her to practice her self-soothing skills and prevent you from placating her at the tiniest cry.

> A 2015 study conducted by scientists in Israel showed just that: Letting baby sleep in her own room significantly improved both infants' and mothers' sleep.

A good time to transition baby into her own room is around two months. At that time, you will be less paranoid about your sleeping baby, and you can actually rest more soundly in your own bedroom.

When your baby becomes a toddler, there will be times when he will want to come to your bed and sleep with you—say, when he's had a nightmare or if he's sick. There is nothing cuter than having your baby or toddler sleep in your bed, on top of you or cradled in

HOW BABIES SLEEP SUCCESS STORY:
Cosleeping to Own Room

Logan's mother, Laura, reached out to me again when he was ten weeks old and thirteen pounds. I'd coached Laura when Logan was just one month old, and his sleep had improved since then. He'd even slept six hours at night a few times. Still, most days and nights were a struggle because Logan had trouble falling asleep during the day and night. At night, he often woke up every hour, and Laura had to nurse him back to sleep. Logan coslept with his parents in the same bed, and often they held Logan for hours during the night, so he could sleep. During the day, he had three to four naps totaling around six hours. Laura was worried that Logan didn't get enough restful sleep, because his arms and legs moved restlessly when he slept, and he "looked unsatisfied," although he didn't cry.

To get Logan back on track, I first advised Laura to get a crib for him and put it in a separate room. She also got a baby monitor so she would feel more comfortable sleeping separately. I counseled Laura on reducing Logan's naps from six to four hours a day, since according to the chart on page 30, Logan was napping too much during the day, which was affecting nighttime sleep. In addition, I guided Laura through Gentle Sleep Training, since Logan was showing signs of readiness (see page 107).

Mom Laura reported back that while it was hard to hear Logan cry, after only a few nights Logan's longest sleep stretch jumped from an average of three hours to a nightly average of five hours! She was thrilled. I advised to continue the sleep training until he was sleeping through the night.

your arm. But be warned: They also think it's great. When they are feeling better and you're ready to get your bedroom back, your little one might have other plans. Evicting a baby or toddler who is used to sleeping with their parents is extremely hard. Most parents give up and let them back in, which can be frustrating when you'd prefer to sleep separately.

You need to decide for yourself what is most important to you, but if you prefer to have your bed to yourself, don't start the habit

Transition from Crib to Bed

When is a good time to transition to a big-kid bed, and how to do it? There is no rush to transition your child to a "real" bed. Kids love routines and consistency and feel cozy and protected in their crib. As long as your child is safe staying in the crib, I recommend leaving her there. Usually around age three, but sometimes much earlier, children start trying to get out of their cribs on their own, which can be unsafe. Once they attempt those "jailbreaks," it is time to transition to a big-kid bed. Before you do it, make sure your child is sleeping well, tired enough in the evening and during the night—otherwise she will be getting out of her bed every five minutes and asking you to entertain her (see step 2 on how to create the ideal schedule). Introduce the idea of transitioning to a big bed a few days before the move, and explain matter-of-factly that she will sleep in a big-kid bed from now on, but that nothing else is changing, and that she will stay in her bed during Night Mode until you or your partner come in in the morning to get her up. If the transition to the big bed wreaks havoc on her bedtime, nighttime sleep, or wake-up time, it means that her schedule has to be reexamined according to step 2. Remember: the bed is not the reason your child is not sleeping well—usually, the schedule is.

of allowing kids to sleep with you. My children have slept with me a handful of times when they were sick, and it felt good having them close by, or rather on top of me. I didn't get much sleep, but I felt like I was helping them get better through the love and care associated with such closeness. However, I insisted on putting them back into the crib the next night, because I did not want them to get used to the mommy pillow.

Siblings

All the core advice in this book was developed when I had my first baby, Leah. When I had my second child, Noah, Leah was two years old. She slept like a champ, but newborn baby Noah, of course, didn't. He was sleeping in our bedroom for the first two months, at which point I was ready to move him to his own bedroom, both for his and our own sakes. His sleep (and ours) improved somewhat, but he kept waking up at night and crying. I was worried Leah would wake up, and I rushed in as fast as I could to nurse Noah each time he cried. Thankfully, Leah rarely woke up.

However, when Noah was around three months and I wanted to sleep train him (see chapters 12 and 13 on how to do it), I knew there would be more crying involved as he learned to self-soothe. The big question was: How do I make sure Leah doesn't wake up, too, leaving me with two sleepless and crying babies? The answer turned out to be easy: separate rooms, white noise, and Night Mode.

Separate Rooms

Ideally each child would be in their own room until everybody is sleep trained. If that's not possible because of space constraints, the one who sleeps better should sleep with you until your other child is sleeping through the night. If you keep the worse sleeper with you—usually the new baby—you will keep waking each other up. Also, sleep training is much easier when baby is not crying right in front of you. Instead, put baby in his own room when you are ready, and put the older kid with you. If everybody sleeps in the same room, white noise and Night Mode are especially important.

White Noise

If the kids are in two separate rooms, get a white noise machine for each room. If the older one sleeps in your room, put a second white noise machine in your bedroom. Turn them on when you put the kids down to sleep. This way, your good sleeper won't wake up when the new baby cries. In a noisy place like a city it will also help drown out traffic noise that might otherwise disturb sleep. If everybody sleeps in the same room, white noise is especially important to prevent waking one another up.

It's also helpful to know that wakings and crying early in the night probably won't disturb the other child as much as later ones. Why? Sleep pressure decreases during the night, as baby or toddler is filling her sleep need (see "Sleep Pressure Makes Us Sleep" on page 28). Her arousal threshold is therefore highest at the beginning of night sleep, and low in the morning before wake-up time. That's when baby's cries are most likely to wake up other children in the house. White noise is especially important in those early morning hours.

Night Mode

No matter how well (or poorly) the new baby sleeps, keep Night Mode in effect in every room the kids are in. This can become very difficult if an older child is woken up by the new baby's crying, or wakes up crying for another reason. Try not to let the older child terminate Night Mode and leave her room. Enlist your partner to take care of one child, if you can, while you placate the other. Strict Night Mode for everyone will prevent weakening rhythms, and this is crucial when it comes to your older child. Remember, if you let her get up too early, it signals to her brain that this, in fact, is the new wake time, and she will be entrained to this new rhythm, even if that means a horrible new wake time of 5 a.m.!

CREATE THE IDEAL LIGHT AND SLEEP ENVIRONMENT
Key Points

★ Establish Day Mode and Night Mode.

★ Use only red light during Night Mode.

★ Make daytime napping less comfortable than nighttime sleeping.

★ Use swaddles, white noise, and other tools only at night to encourage baby to sleep through the night.

★ Figure out a sleeping arrangement that works for your family.

Step 2: Create the Ideal Sleep and Nap Schedule

Now you're an expert on creating an ideal sleep environment for baby. But what about schedules and routines? When are we supposed to feed baby, and when is she supposed to sleep? Or should we follow our baby's cues to decide? Thankfully, science can help us figure out those crucial questions.

You learned in "The Science of Sleep" that our internal clock is very precise, which means that the more aligned you are with your endogenous rhythm, the easier it will be to go to bed and wake up every day. In plain English, this means: do everything at the same time every day, and don't make any exceptions. You want to establish consistent times for nighttime sleep, naps, and feedings. In addition, you can add specific times when you go out every day, play, or do other activities. In the next chapters you will learn how to establish and maintain the different elements of baby's schedule—feeds, bed and wake times, naps and routines from the day he is born.

Chapter 8

Schedules

Multiple studies show that putting babies on a schedule helps them cry less and helps parents feel less overwhelmed. One of the main questions parents have is how to get their baby on a schedule—and from what age that is even possible.

Newborns

In the very beginning, we are told in the hospital or by our pediatrician to nurse on demand, and that the newborn should wake up every two hours to nurse, and maybe have one three-to-four-hour stretch of sleep during the night.

Usually doctors recommend waking babies up at night after four hours to nurse them, until they have regained their birth weight (unless they are preemies, in which case the doctor will give you a different goal weight). When born, babies transition from constant feeding through mom's blood supply in utero to intermittent milk feeding, and initially lose weight in the process. It's important to facilitate sufficient hydration and calories until babies regain their birth weight. That generally happens between one week and one month after your baby is born. Until then, wake baby up after four hours of sleep at night, and feed her every two hours during the day.

Once baby regains his birth weight, it's usually okay to let him sleep at night. Blissful! This was pretty much the progression with my first baby, Leah. After two weeks she had regained her birth weight, and slept through the night from then on.

Baby number two was an entirely different story. When our son, Noah, was born, he nursed every fifteen minutes for the first twenty-four hours, and then every half hour for the next forty-eight hours. He would nurse for just a few minutes, never emptying even one breast, and fall asleep for a short while, then wake up hungry again. Repeat. After three days of this madness I asked my doula (a birth and newborn helper) what to do, and she told me he should nurse every two hours and sleep in between. So I made him do just that. I kept him awake during feedings by undressing him and blowing air on him when he was falling asleep, and that way he ate more and was able to sleep for longer stretches between feedings. After only two feedings like this we were on the every-two-hour schedule, which made my life much more sane, because now I was able to catch up on sleep a little when he was sleeping—a luxury that is impossible when the baby feeds every fifteen to thirty minutes.

> Newborns should feed every two hours and sleep in between.

This goes to show that, while at that stage we can't yet impose any rhythm on the baby, even newborns respond to incentives to feed and sleep when we would like them to.

To repeat: Newborns should feed every two hours and sleep in between. At night, one four-hour stretch is allowed. To make sleepy babies stay awake and nurse longer to fill them up, undress them, get a cold wet cloth, and touch them a little, or blow air at them.

Why Schedules Are Important

Between baby-led chaos and strict routines that ignore baby's cues, there is a natural way to establish routines for baby and yourself. Baby-led feeding and sleeping without gentle reinforcement and transition to a routine is problematic because baby has no clue yet as to what time of day it is—and more importantly, she doesn't know herself well enough yet to understand her own needs. She might be upset but not know why. It might be because she is hungry, it might be because she is tired, it might be for another reason we will never know. Worse, if there is no routine, we will have to try all possibilities each time—feed her, change her, try to put her down—which is exhausting for both you and the baby. By the time you figure out what she needs she might have already cried for twenty minutes and now be much harder to console.

By establishing feeding and sleeping routines, you and your baby will both learn to understand what the baby needs at certain times. You and the baby will learn that he is upset just before nap time because he is tired, and that going to sleep will make him feel better. You and your baby will understand that he is cranky at 10 a.m. because he is hungry, and that getting a bottle or being nursed will help. Of course, there will still be times when baby is upset and cries without it being clear why this is the case. But those times will be dramatically reduced, because usually the baby's needs will be met by the routines you established.

> By establishing feeding and sleeping routines, you and your baby will both learn to understand what the baby needs at certain times.

What other advantages are there to scheduled over random feeding and naps? Less stress, less crying, more freedom. Baby will quickly learn when it is time to feed and not expect food at other times. He will be calmer overall, because his body is more organized. For you, the schedule simplifies life significantly. If an hour has passed since a feed and baby is fussy, you know not to feed him, but to soothe him in another way, because he cannot be hungry. If it's just before a scheduled feed and he's fussy, you know he's hungry and will start your prefeeding routine, be it picking him up and carrying him around or changing his diaper and doing some tummy time.

For you, a schedule means you can actually get your life back a little bit, because now you're able to plan your day a bit better. You know you can work, or see a doctor, or meet a friend for coffee at 11:30 a.m. because your baby will be fed and happy for another two hours. Amazing!

> For you, a schedule means you can actually get your life back a little bit, because now you're able to plan your day a bit better.

So how do we accomplish a feeding and nap schedule? Even in the first weeks of life, when baby eats very often, you can begin to establish certain feeding times (see "Sample Schedules for Babies from 0–5 Months" on page 79). First set up a fixed time for the last feed before bedtime, and then add the first one in the morning.

Setting Bedtime and Morning Wake Time

The beauty of this program is that you get to choose the sleep and wake schedule that works for you. In this way, How Babies Sleep differs from all other sleep training advice. From the very start, figure out what your desired schedule is and entrain baby to align her sleep cycle to yours. Putting her down too early will result in a baby who wakes up too early, because she can sleep only so many hours at a time, and stay only so long in Night Mode. If your baby sleeps at most five hours at a time, and you put her down at 7 p.m., she will wake up at midnight and not sleep as long or well after. Unless you want to go to bed at 7 p.m., baby's schedule will be misaligned with yours.

The best way to set appropriate bed and wake times is to work backward from your desired wake time. This makes sense for most parents who eventually have to go back to work, or who have other kids who get up at a particular time. For example, if your goal is an 8 a.m. wake time, and you'd like to go to bed at 11 p.m., between 11 p.m. and 8 a.m. are the core Night Mode hours. Baby's last feed would be before that, at 10:30 p.m., and it should be in Night Mode, to signal to baby that it's now time to sleep. Be-

> The best way to set appropriate bed and wake times is to work backward from your desired wake time.

fore that you will have a whole night routine that will entrain baby to anticipate bedtime (see page 90 for a sample bedtime routine).

If baby nurses multiple times during the night and you're up for hours during that time, you might want to add a buffer at the start or end of the night so you can get enough rest. If baby nurses three times during the night and it takes forty minutes each time to feed, change diapers, and soothe, you could add 3 × 40 minutes = 2 hours at the start of the night to get enough sleep. Last feed would be 8:30 p.m. and bedtime 9 p.m. Alternatively, you can add one hour at night and one hour in the morning. Each time baby drops a night feed, you can adjust bed and wake times.

This whole process can be tricky if baby's night sleep and number of night feedings are still highly variable, typically in the first two months. The solution is to pick bed and wake times that give you enough rest, and keep Night Mode for that whole time. Baby will quickly learn that this is the time to sleep. Even if she still needs to feed frequently, she will go back to sleep quickly after feeding and not expect daytime playing and activities. The key is to keep strict Night Mode until your designated wake time.

Let's go through the process of creating a schedule for a one-week-old newborn together.

Step 1: Determine your desired wake-up time. Let's say it's 7 a.m.

Step 2: Determine how much time in total you are awake at night. Let's say one hour.

Step 3: Look at the baby sleep chart on page 30 and find your baby's age. At one week, she should sleep nine hours at night (plus night wakings to feed).

Step 4: Calculate bedtime: your desired wake time minus baby's total nighttime sleep time. That's 7 a.m. – 9 hours = 10 p.m. Because of the nighttime wakings, add an hour of buffer at the beginning of the night, so bedtime is 9 p.m. Bedtime routine, including nursing or feeding, starts at least 30 minutes earlier, at 8:30 p.m.

Your schedule: Night Mode begins at 8:30 p.m., feed, bedtime 9 p.m., wake time 7 a.m.

Establishing a Daytime Feeding and Nap Schedule

Babies are born with an internal clock, as you now know, but that clock is neither internally nor externally aligned yet—their schedule is erratic. It's neither possible nor helpful to impose a strict sleep schedule on newborns, but it is useful to establish a feeding schedule, as well as keep constant bed and wake times. For babies up to one month old, try to keep the feedings constant and see what works best for naps, because baby will be tired soon after a feed.

If you want to go to bed at 10:30 p.m. and get up at 8 a.m., have the last scheduled feed at 10 p.m., and nurse your baby at 8 a.m., no matter how often you nursed during the night, or when the previous feed was. You want to establish those feeds as zeitgebers and stick to them. Eventually, you will add set times for all the other feeds. You can do this even with the two-hour newborn schedule,

Newborn–8 weeks	
9:00 AM	**Wake and Feed**
10:00 AM	Nap (30-60 minutes)
11:00 AM	Wake and Feed
12:30 PM	Nap (30-60 minutes)
1:30 PM	Wake and Feed
3:30 PM	Nap (30-60 minutes)
4:30 PM	Wake and Feed
6:00 PM	Nap (30-60 minutes)
6:30 PM	Wake and Feed
7:30 PM	Catnap (20-30 minutes)
8:00 PM	Wake and Feed
9:00 PM	Catnap (20-30 minutes)
10:00 PM	**Bedtime Routine**
10:30 PM	**Feed and Sleep**

+ Nighttime feedings in night mode
Bold denotes fixed times

2-Month-Old Baby	
8:30 AM	Wake and Feed
10:30 AM	Nap
11:30 AM	Wake
12:00 PM	Feed
1:30 PM	Nap
3:30 PM	Wake
4:00 PM	Feed
5:30 PM	Nap
6:30 PM	Wake and Feed
8:30 PM	Feed and Nap
9:30 PM	Wake
10:15 PM	Start Bedtime Routine
10:30 PM	Bath
10:45 PM	Feed and Sleep

+ Nighttime feedings in night mode

3-Month-Old Baby	
8:30 AM	Wake and Feed
10:30 AM	Nap
11:30 AM	Wake
12:00 PM	Feed
2:00 PM	Nap
3:30 PM	Wake and Feed
6:00 PM	Feed
6:15 PM	Nap
7:00 PM	Wake
8:00 PM	Feed
9:15 PM	Start bedtime routine
9:30 PM	Bath
9:45 PM	Feed and Sleep

+ Nighttime feedings in night mode

5-Month-Old Baby	
8:00 AM	Wake and Feed
10:30 AM	Nap
11:15 AM	Wake
12:00 PM	Feed
2:00 PM	Nap
3:30 PM	Wake and Feed
6:00 PM	Feed and Nap
6:45 PM	Wake
8:00 PM	Feed
8:30 PM	Bedtime Routine
8:45 PM	Bath
9:15 PM	Feed and Sleep

+ Nighttime feedings in night mode

Sample Schedules for Babies from 0–5 Months
While newborns sleep most of the time, as baby gets a little older she will be awake for longer stretches of time after feedings. Also, the number of naps will decrease. You will notice a pattern emerging, like: feed, stay awake for an hour, sleep for an hour or two. Take note of those patterns and incorporate them into your schedule. Why do babies sleep so much when they are born? While there is no definitive answer to this question, we can understand baby's frequent sleeps in the context of sleep pressure (see page 28).

but it really starts making sense when you transition to bigger intervals, like feeding every two and a half to three hours. Exactly when this happens depends on your baby and, in particular, her weight gain. Every baby is different, and you will naturally respect your baby's needs, because she will show you she's hungry by crying, rooting, and putting her hand in her mouth. If baby still needs to nurse every two hours, then just do it. When she is big enough to go for three hours without food, just fill in the feeding times during the day starting with your established wake time and ending with your established bedtime.

Just like sleep training, naps, and cosleeping, feeding babies is another hot-button topic in the parenting and pediatric communities. Parents disagree on whether to feed babies on demand or according to a schedule. While I don't recommend imposing a strict schedule on a newborn, it's worth noting that preterm babies who are hospitalized in neonatal infant care units (NICUs) until they are mature enough to be released home are fed on a three-hour schedule long before they are full term, depending on their weight. At home, we feed newborns during the day around every two hours, which usually can be stretched to every three hours by two months.

Usually, babies are more tired in the morning than the evening and will go down for the next nap sooner after first waking in the morning. The more feedings and naps you can keep the same, the easier it will be for both of you.

In the evening, babies are often hungrier and need to feed more frequently, which might even result in constant nursing in very young babies, called cluster feeding. This is useful because it fills them up for the night and helps them sleep longer (see page 85).

How do you know what schedule works for your baby? Once babies have regained their birth weight, they should be able to last for two hours between feeds. This interval will slowly grow. If you consistently see baby still happy or sleeping two hours

> Once babies have regained their birth weight, they should be able to last for two hours between feeds.

HOW BABIES SLEEP SUCCESS STORY:
Schedule for a Newborn

Remember Laura and Logan from pages 44 and 65? When Laura first reached out to me, Logan was a month old and Laura was dead tired because she had barely slept since he was born. What's worse, she didn't even know what was day and what was night anymore—it had all become a blur, because Logan was often up every thirty minutes and cried, although he also managed to sleep for four hours straight at night a few times.

To start, I helped Laura establish a schedule. Her preferred wake time was 7 a.m., and she needed eight hours of sleep to feel okay. Because of Logan's frequent night wakings, we needed to add buffer time to Night Mode, so that Laura could get enough sleep at night. We established that Logan's bedtime should be 10 p.m. and wake time 8 a.m., with strict Night Mode between these hours. The extra hour in the morning would help Laura sleep a little longer to make up for lost sleep during the night. The bedtime was a late 10 p.m. because that's when Logan's longest sleep stretch—four hours—happened. It started when Laura went to bed, so she could get a solid four-hour stretch of sleep before he woke up again. Naps should be unrestricted at this age; however, I instructed Laura to avoid swaddling Logan during the day or making it too dark for naps, and that she shouldn't use white noise or be too quiet around him. We wanted Logan to get adequate sleep during the day so that he wasn't overtired, but also to have enough sleep pressure to sleep longer overnight. I told Laura to consult the baby sleep chart (page 30) as Logan grows and start restricting his napping by waking him up gently if he exceeded recommended nap durations. Establishing a sleep schedule was immensely helpful for mom and baby—Laura reported getting more sleep and feeling more like her old self.

after a feed, try extending the interval to two hours and fifteen minutes or two and a half hours. If that works, stick to it until the same thing happens and baby shows you he can go longer between feeds. Look at the table on page 79 for sample schedules for babies of different ages. Those are almost the exact schedules we used for both our babies.

Why Schedule Naps?

What's the advantage of scheduling naps versus letting baby decide when to sleep? A lack of structure will cause difficulties for baby and parents. Baby will be somewhat tired around certain times of day, but if you don't help him recognize his fatigue and put him down at predictable times, he will be cranky for hours and not know what to do. Sometimes he will be tired enough to pass out, sometimes he won't, and you will have one unhappy baby on your hands. It's much better to help baby organize his day by creating a nap schedule. This way there won't be any surprises for baby, and he will learn that when he feels tired, he needs to sleep.

Scientists believe that babies' sleep pressure rises much faster (see "Sleep Pressure Makes Us Sleep" on page 28) than adults', which explains why they have to sleep so frequently. This fits well with our observations. Newborns wake up only to feed, falling asleep quickly thereafter. As baby gets older, she can remain more alert, taking in her surroundings and interacting with them more. Naps are spaced farther apart as the baby grows.

When you're ready to set scheduled feeding times, the nap times will follow naturally. The interval between naps is very small in a newborn. Baby sleeps most of the time and wakes up only to feed. After a few days, he starts to be awake for a while after each feed. When the interval approaches two-plus hours, you can start reinforcing the pattern by playing with him a little before you put him down or feed him.

It's very common for parents to feel like they should feed the baby immediately after every nap, especially since that's often what needs to happen for newborns, who feed every two hours. But this is not necessary as the baby gets older. Whether baby feeds before, after, or right between naps is irrelevant. The only time when feeding should directly precede sleep is at bedtime, because it fills baby up, calms her, and transitions her into night sleep. During the day, naps and feeding can be disjointed, as sleep need and hunger are not correlated.

For example, at three months, baby is awake for two to two and a half hours between naps, but feeds can already be three to three and a half hours apart. Also, the nap intervals increase during the day, while the feeding intervals decrease. Baby is most tired in the morning and will stay awake longer and longer between naps as the day goes by. Conversely, babies tend to be hungrier in the evening and feed more often. For that reason, feeding doesn't need to coincide with the start or end of the nap. See table on page 79 for examples of schedules for different ages.

To avoid the human pacifier trap of constant nursing (see page 86), enlist help if possible. Daddy, a grandparent, a friend, a babysitter, or a nanny can take baby out for a walk when it's nap time. Baby will sleep without wanting to nurse, and if this happens consistently at the same time every day, it will reinforce this particular nap time.

HOW BABIES SLEEP SUCCESS STORY:
Schedule for a 5-month-old

Katie contacted me for help with her five-month-old baby, Ava. Ava was born at five and a half pounds, and at five months weighed twelve pounds. She didn't sleep through the night, but would wake up multiple times. She also got up at 5 a.m.—way too early for her parents. Her bedtime routine started at 6:15 p.m., and mom or dad usually rocked her to sleep. Ava woke up at 11 p.m. and 3 a.m., and Katie usually nursed her back to sleep. Katie told me Ava's sleep was very erratic and that only on rare occasions had Ava slept for eight hours straight. Ava's napping was random. On average, Ava had three or four naps a day, and the total daytime sleep varied from three to four hours total.

There were many things we could improve to help Ava sleep longer at night. First, I helped Katie adjust Ava's room to optimize sleep—she got a red lamp and blackout shades. Then we helped get Ava on a nap and feeding schedule. Katie reviewed the baby sleep chart (page 30) and together we developed a schedule that works for everyone.

According to the chart, five-month-olds sleep an average of ten and a half hours at night, which means for a desired wake-up time of 7 a.m., bedtime should be no earlier than 8:30 p.m.—Ava's 6:15 p.m. bedtime was way too early. Young babies have one long sleep stretch at the start of the night, and you want that to start close to your own bedtime, so that you can get some decent sleep.

Katie created a bedtime routine that started at 8 p.m. and included a bath, a book, a song, and nursing. I explained to Katie why it was important to put her baby down in her crib while awake, instead of nursing her to sleep, to help her learn how to self-soothe.

In addition to these changes, Katie and I worked on creating a nap schedule. Most five-month-olds sleep about two and a half hours during the day, and usually transition from three to two naps around that age. We transitioned Ava slowly to a consistent three-nap schedule, where she sleeps forty-five minutes in the morning, one hour after lunch, and forty-five minutes in the afternoon. It's very much okay to wake Ava up if she sleeps too long, and if she's a little cranky, her parents can distract her with a toy, or Katie can nurse her a little to placate her.

These changes alone made a major difference for Katie and Ava! Next we worked on Gentle Sleep Training (page 110), and after a short period of time, Ava's sleep dramatically improved and the whole family got some much-needed rest.

Cluster Feeding in the Evening

Between 7 p.m. and bedtime, baby will likely not sleep much, and that's okay, because after this stretch of wakefulness he will go down for the night. Babies are often fussy during this "witching hour" because they are exhausted from the day. Sleep scientists actually believe the reason babies are often cranky in the evening is because their sleep rhythm hasn't matured yet. As adults, we are usually able to maintain reasonable wakefulness until we almost suddenly get very tired and conk out. In babies, toward the evening, sleep pressure is high, even though it's not time to sleep yet. That's why they are so cranky during these hours before bedtime. They often need extra attention and soothing, which can be exhausting, and might also feed more frequently or even cluster feed to prepare for their long stretch of sleep.

Many parents find themselves exhausted and worn out by this

point in the day, and it can be trying to manage everything at once. Keep reading for some good ways to minimize fussiness and soothe your baby during the witching hour. And know that after this fussy time, you will do your bedtime routine and baby will go down for her longest stretch of the night.

The Human Pacifier Trap

For nursing mothers, it can be difficult to see a fussy baby and not give him the breast, because it is the easiest way to calm him. The problem with this approach is that it leads to nonstop nursing and a baby who gets used to the constant availability of the breast. If offered the breast too often, the baby will not eat a full meal but only suckle a little, and get hungry again soon after. This is exhausting for both parents and baby, so try to remain steadfast and not offer the breast until it's feeding time again, whether it's two, two and a half, or three hours after your last feed, depending on your schedule. Remember that newborns need to feed every two hours, and that you'll want to include more frequent feeds during the witching hour when baby is cluster feeding in the evening before bedtime (see the sample schedule on page 79).

I personally found it very difficult to not nurse Leah and Noah whenever they got fussy, and it was only with the help of the nanny and my going back to work that we were able to break the habit of constant snacking. Therefore, if possible, enlist help—ask your partner, a family member, or a babysitter to take the baby, if that's available to you.

If your baby is fussy before her feed or nap time, calm her in another way; for example, rock her or go out for a walk in the stroller. Play with her on the floor, give her a bath, sing to her, or listen to music. In addition to creating a feeding and sleeping schedule, it is helpful to create a plan, as in: every day we'll do tummy time at

5 p.m., go for a walk at 6 p.m., and listen to music at 7 p.m. (see chapter 9). Structuring your day like this sounds over-the-top, but it helps both you and baby: you know what to do next, and baby gets habituated, or, in chronobiology terms, entrained to certain things happening at certain times, which will help her cope with the unease of feeling tired but not tired enough to sleep.

If baby is fussy and it is time to sleep, use rocking, swaddling, electric swing, or other sleep aids discussed on page 57 to help baby fall asleep. Again, try to start using the same aids for the same naps, to create routines for yourself and baby.

HOW BABIES SLEEP SUCCESS STORY:
The Human Pacifier Trap

Mom Natalia and dad Amir were desperate. Their six-month-old, Lucas, was a happy baby, except when it came to sleeping at night. The biggest problem was that Lucas refused to sleep at night unless mom lay next to him and nursed him, effectively turning Natalia into a human pacifier. If she dared to remove herself and her breast from Lucas, he would wake up after twenty minutes and demand her return. It was exhausting. Napping was also difficult, and Lucas slept only when he was bounced in the carrier by mom or dad. If put down in the crib by himself, whether during the day or at night, he would immediately start screaming.

To get out of the human pacifier trap, I walked Natalia and Amir through the basic How Babies Sleep method. They moved Lucas to a separate room and got blackout shades and a red light. Then we tackled his sleep schedule. He had been waking up between 7 and 7:30 a.m. and taking three naps of an hour each, then going to bed at 7 p.m. We restricted his naps to a total of two and a half hours and moved bedtime to 8:30 p.m. (see page 93 on the ideal nap schedule).

The hardest part of breaking this pattern was getting him to sleep overnight. We needed to retrain Lucas to accept sleeping on his own, using self-soothing instead of parental soothing to fall and stay asleep. This is really hard, especially for a six-month-old, at which age he remembers how nice it feels to sleep with his mommy right next to him. He will protest, and his parents have to stand it—a little bit. I introduced the science behind my Gentle Sleep Training (page 110) to Natalia and Amir, and we made the plan to not nurse Lucas more frequently than every four hours at night.

Two weeks later, when I checked in with Natalia and Amir, they confessed that sleep training wasn't going that well. Their apartment was under construction, therefore both kids were sleeping in their parents' room, which prevented getting started on Gentle Sleep Training. A month and many sleepless nights later, Natalia found the inner strength to start implementing my program. They evicted the baby from their bedroom, and Natalia stopped immediately nursing when Lucas started crying at night. After only two nights a miracle happened: while Lucas still sometimes woke up and cried, his sleep jumped from waking up every hour to waking up every four to five hours, and sometimes he even put himself back to sleep. Yay!

Chapter 9

Routines

The easiest way to establish scheduled events like going to bed at night is to come up with a routine, which you will repeat every day. Babies and adults thrive on behavioral sequences that are constant from day to day. You probably know that from your own experience: there is something pleasant and reassuring about knowing what will happen next. In the morning you get up, shower, brush your teeth, get dressed, and drink a coffee, and the expectation of this order of events has a soothing quality to it. It's no different for babies. Knowing what will happen next makes them calmer and happier.

Bedtime Routine

The most important task is establishing a bedtime routine, and then sticking to it. Every. Single. Day. Come up with a set of things you do every night before you put baby down. This might look something like this:

PRE-NIGHT MODE
- Give baby a massage.
- Give baby a bath.
- Carry baby to the nursery.

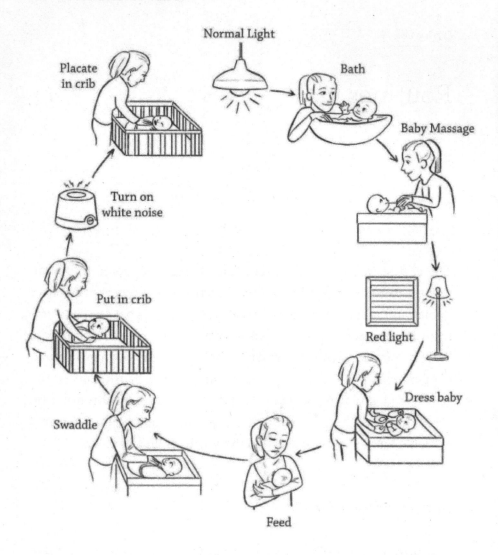

Normal Light

Placate
in crib

Bath

Baby Massage

Turn on
white noise

Red light

Put in crib

Dress baby

Swaddle

Feed

Bedtime Routine
It helps baby to transition to sleep if she experiences the same chain of events
every night before bed. You don't have to incorporate every element shown
here, and can instead use other actions, like reading a book or singing a song.
It's important to do the same things every night, so baby knows what to expect. The only nonnegotiable item is the light: once Night Mode begins, keep
baby's room dark with blackout shades, and only use red light from then on,
and during the night.

NIGHT MODE

- From now on no more talking, only whispering. Tell baby he's tired and now it's time to go to sleep.
- Prepare bedroom/nursery and diaper-changing area before you come in with baby so that shades are shut, lights are off, and red lamp is on.
- Change baby.
- Nurse baby or give a bottle.
- Swaddle baby (I usually swaddled mine between the first and second breasts, because that way they were all ready to be put in the crib after eating).
- Put baby down in the crib.
- Turn on white noise.
- If baby cries, rock her bassinet or stroke her in the crib. Try to avoid picking her up. If she won't settle and you have to pick her up, avoid nursing or feeding her.

DURING THE NIGHT

- Don't nurse or feed until it's feeding time again.
- Nurse or feed in a dedicated spot in his bedroom, keep the swaddle on, and don't talk. Keep the room quiet and dark, with only the red light on.
- If baby is older than four months or weighs more than eleven pounds, try Gentle Sleep Training (page 110).

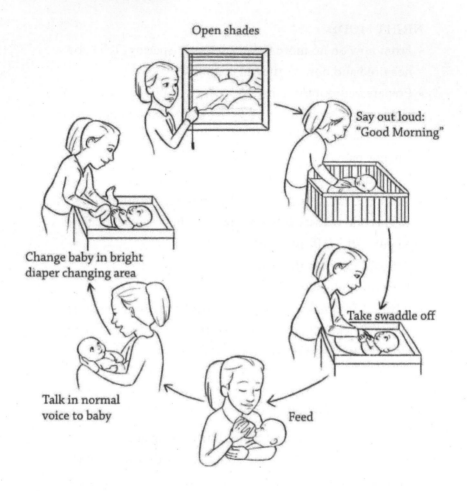

Open shades

Say out loud: "Good Morning"

Take swaddle off

Feed

Change baby in bright diaper changing area

Talk in normal voice to baby

Morning Routine

Every morning when it's your desired wake-up time, go into baby's room, open the shades, and say "Good morning" in a loud voice. Proceed by taking baby's swaddle off, feeding him, and changing him, all while talking to him in a normal daytime voice. Make it clear—the day starts now!

Chapter 10

Naps

We learned in chapter 6 about Day and Night Modes, and how we want to make Night Mode as conducive to long stretches of sleep as possible. During the day we do the opposite. Yes, naps are necessary, but we don't want baby to nap all day.

So how much should baby nap, and how much is too much? Getting baby on a nap and feeding schedule will help you structure your days and produce a calmer, happier baby (and parents!). Maintaining clear Day and Night Modes will help baby to learn that nighttime is for sleeping and daytime is for napping. He will still wake up to feed at night in the early months but will go straight back to sleep after, without much or any soothing required. While these are major accomplishments, those nighttime feedings, however short and easy they are, will still present a challenge to the parent who has to get up (typically the mother, especially if she is nursing). Feeds during the first few hours of mother's sleep are particularly disruptive for truly restorative sleep. The best thing to do is to limit naps during the day and start Gentle Sleep Training when baby is ready.

Your baby has a total daily sleep need that steadily decreases as she gets older. To better understand your baby's sleep patterns, start logging her sleep now. You can use old-fashioned pen and paper or one of the many baby tracker apps for smartphones. Once you have a sense of her schedule, compare it to the chart on page 30. Is your baby napping too long? Or going to bed too early at night? If so, adjust her naps and bedtime accordingly. Instead of logging baby's sleep, you can also use our Kulala baby sleep app (see page 193 and the last page) to create a customized schedule for your baby.

Sometimes parents are confused because their baby doesn't fit squarely into the chart: he is sleeping less than the average baby his age. What does that mean? It means your baby is advanced in terms of his sleep development! My chart reflects global averages for sleep, and most babies fit well into those norms. However, some babies need more sleep, and others need less. The good news is that no matter where your baby starts out, the overall trend is the same: newborns sleep a lot, and they will sleep less as they get older.

If your baby sleeps less than the average baby, simply look at the bar for an older baby in the chart, starting with the next age group and going down from there until you find one that matches. Use that age as a point of reference to determine nighttime and daytime sleep durations. For example: Your six-month-old already only sleeps twelve and a half hours total per day, and naps only two hours. In contrast, the chart says six-month-olds sleep thirteen hours total, and nap two and a half hours. Your baby is an advanced sleeper, so find the age corresponding to your baby's total sleep, which is twelve months old. Twelve-month-olds sleep eleven hours at night and one and a half hours during the day, so try to use those numbers to establish a schedule for your baby. This means cutting down daytime sleep by one hour so as to increase nighttime sleep from ten straight hours to eleven.

Reducing Daytime Sleep

Sleep is vital for babies, and parents have a lot of anxiety over whether baby is getting enough sleep and sleeping at the right time. This is compounded by the fact that there are common misconceptions about naps that can get in the way of effective sleep training, such as:

- Sleep begets sleep: baby needs to sleep a lot during the day to be able to sleep well at night.
- We need to do everything in our power to help baby nap as much as possible.
- Don't wake a sleeping baby.

The truth is that all of these opinions are scientifically wrong, and following them will make it harder to get your baby to sleep through the night. In fact, research has shown that duration of daytime sleep is *inversely* correlated with nighttime sleep in young children—that means too much napping will lead to sleepless nights.

> Research has shown that duration of daytime sleep is *inversely* correlated with nighttime sleep in young children—that means too much napping will lead to sleepless nights.

I learned this the hard way. When Leah was born, my husband and I were taught how to swaddle her. Seeing how useful it was to calm her down when she was crying, and how much it comforted her, we used swaddles all the time. For the first six weeks we swaddled her for all naps and during nighttime sleep. While we were very lucky in that Leah slept for six or seven hours at night, starting from around two weeks of age, getting her down to sleep at night was a nightmare. As soon as I tried to put her down in the evening, around 9 p.m. (too early, in hindsight), she would start crying and I had to pick her up and rock her in my arms. When she calmed down and seemed to fall asleep, I would put her back in her crib. As soon as she hit the crib, she would start crying hysterically again, and I had to pick her up again, carry her around, shush her, rock her in my arms, etc. This went on for more than three hours, every night for three weeks.

One day, when she was around five weeks old, I had an idea. I stopped swaddling her during the day, which meant that it was a little bit harder for her to go to sleep during her naps. It meant I had to soothe her more when she was tired and cranky to help her go to sleep during the day. Importantly, it also meant that she woke up earlier from naps, and napped less in total, because her flailing arms and sleep twitching would wake her up. The result? That night she went to bed without crying, and the three-hour crying spells subsided forever. The swaddles were encouraging her to sleep too much during the day, and that prevented her from being tired enough when bedtime came around—her sleep pressure was too low. What I gave up in daytime napping I gained in the evening. It seemed like a good trade to me!

Daytime naps are a big point of contention in the parenting and parenting-advice communities. New parents are warned to never wake a sleeping baby. Many moms are confused about naps and whether they affect how well baby sleeps at night. Science has a clear answer to that question. How much we sleep at night depends on our sleep pressure, and that sleep pressure is lessened by sleep, in particular naps. Assuming you aren't already sleep deprived, if you take a two-hour nap during the day, you won't be as tired in the evening and might have trouble falling asleep at bedtime. That long nap will lower your sleep pressure. It has been shown that there is a clear relationship between number of naps, nap duration, and nighttime sleep in small children.

> Babies who sleep more during the day go to bed later at night and sleep less during the night.

Babies who sleep more during the day go to bed later at night and sleep less during the night. It's really logical, and what it means for your baby is that you might have to restrict daytime napping. Of course, this isn't always what parents want to hear, because naps are the only times during the day when mom and dad have a chance to get anything done, whether that's taking a shower, eating, running errands, or taking their own nap. I'm not going to lie—to this day I hate waking my babies up from their blissful sleep (and I have had to endure harsh words from our first nanny, who believed it's unhealthy for Leah if I don't let her sleep). The choice is yours: let them sleep during the day and be up at night, or vice versa. I suspect you'll opt for the latter, and if you do, the solution is very clear: cut their naps!

Shortening naps is also crucial before you start sleep training. Sleep training will not work or will be very hard if baby's nighttime sleep is supposed to

> The choice is yours: let them sleep during the day and be up at night, or vice versa.

be longer than her sleep need permits. Therefore, it's important to first figure out how many hours baby can sleep at night and how to maximize daytime wakefulness with minimal napping, before attempting to drop nighttime feedings.

How to Shorten Daytime Naps

Examine the baby sleep chart (page 30) and compare the numbers to your baby. If she sleeps too much during the day, shorten nap times so that the total amount of sleep during the day matches the chart. You don't have to do anything radical, but if, for example, you are settled in a schedule where baby has three two-hour naps during the day but should only be sleeping five hours during the day according to the baby sleep chart, you need to cut one hour in total, or twenty minutes off each nap for example. Once you reduce the daytime sleeping by enough time, baby will be more tired at night, which will help him sleep longer.

How to get them to sleep less during naps? The easiest way is to reduce sleep aids (see page 57), as suggested in chapter 7. If you use swaddling and white noise at night, don't use them during the day.

If you use a swing and nap time is over, turn the swing off to prevent baby from being rocked to sleep indefinitely. If he sleeps in a stroller and motion makes him sleepy, stop walking around with the stroller. If baby loves sleeping on his tummy, put him on his back. (The American Academy of Pediatrics cautions against tummy sleeping, as explained on page 54.) If baby keeps sleeping despite these changes, don't be afraid to wake him by picking him up. Letting sleeping babies lie is not good advice in this context. Your baby will be just fine if you wake him, and will likely sleep better at night. If baby is cranky when you wake him up, a good strategy is to quickly distract him by feeding him or showing him something interesting, like a toy or something out the window.

Another aspect of cutting daytime sleep is prolonging the time baby spends awake between naps. When you shorten nap durations and baby wakes up from her nap earlier than before, she might feel tired earlier, before the next nap time starts. Try to gently stretch the period between naps by entertaining baby. Remember, it's fine for her to be awake a little longer than before, like thirty to forty-five minutes. Of course, if you feel like baby is dead tired and needs to nap, put her down.

What do you do if your baby has taken his allotted nap hours and it's still three hours till bedtime proper? It's okay to let baby take a fourth catnap in the evening, especially in the early days when he cannot stay awake for very long yet (see page 79 for example schedules). Don't let him sleep for too long, though; usually thirty to forty minutes will be enough.

As a rule of thumb, try cutting daytime sleep by 20 percent and see if it helps with nighttime sleep. Closely monitor baby's reaction during the day and night to those changes. You need to find the fine line of minimal daytime naps that still produce a mostly happy, if occasionally cranky because tired baby. If you see an improvement at first but her sleep worsens after a while, you can reduce daytime naps even further. This is a constant process of monitoring baby's

HOW BABIES SLEEP SUCCESS STORY:
Shortening Naps

Mom Amber wanted help with three-month-old baby Mason's sleep, because his nighttime sleep was erratic: sometimes he would sleep six hours in a stretch and once even seven hours, but sometimes he would wake up after only one and a half hours of sleeping, demanding to be fed. Yet he didn't seem very hungry at those times, and fell asleep while nursing. He was napping around four and a half hours a day.

In addition to making key changes to the light settings in the nursery to help entrain Mason to a better sleep schedule, we had to shorten his naps to three and a half hours total, which is the average for children his age. We transitioned him from four naps to three, with respective durations of one hour, one and a half hours, and then one hour again.

Amber called me up a few days later and happily told me that Mason's sleep had improved practically overnight, and he was now sleeping 6-hour stretches most nights.

sleep and adjusting nap durations and times, because her total daily sleep need is gradually decreasing and to sleep at night she needs to sleep less during the day. Keep referencing the baby sleep chart (page 30) to compare your baby's total sleep and daytime sleep to her age group and adjust accordingly. Another tool is our Kulala baby sleep app, which creates customized schedules for babies based on the methods described in this book; see page 193 and the last page for more information.

Chapter 11

Repetition and Flexibility

As you've learned, every action and behavior either reinforces or disrupts the circadian rhythm. Understanding this is very important, because it's not always easy to stick to the schedule when your baby seems to want to sleep/wake/feed at other times. But it's very important to do so. Remember, giving in is not just a one-off event, but actually steers the ship in the wrong direction, making it harder for baby to sleep through the night.

> Every action and behavior either reinforces or disrupts the circadian rhythm.

I think this realization helped me the most during the tough phases of sleep training: that any exception, any deviation from our schedule would weaken baby's rhythm, and even put him on the path to a different rhythm that didn't work with ours. Once you understand this, you will be able to stick to the sleep and wake times, and to all the routines that go along with them. Research supports that minimal variability in daily schedules is highly beneficial to our health—and baby's sleep. A national poll in 2009 conducted by researchers from different US institutions, including Brown University and the University of Michigan, found that children who don't have a consistent bedtime routine sleep worse at night than children who do the same steps at bedtime every night. Furthermore, one of the most successful interventions to decrease baby's crying is creating daily feeding and sleep schedules.

While you will need to be quite strict in sticking to Day and Night Modes and the daily feeding and sleep schedule, you will also need to stay in tune with your baby and how the schedule is working for her. If something consistently doesn't work, try adjusting it. As I said in the very beginning of this book, trust your intuition above all. All aspects of How Babies Sleep are set yet movable parts. Your baby is growing and changing, and has growth spurts, teething pains, and all other kinds of events and processes going on in her little body that need constant observation, because they can affect how much sleep she needs.

There are two overarching trends that will guide you: As baby grows, he will feed less frequently and therefore be able to sleep longer at night, and his total twenty-four-hour sleep need will decrease. Keep those two trends in mind when adjusting bedtime, nap times, and feeding times. Rest assured that reinforcing patterns and repeating routines at certain times during the day will work thanks to baby's biology: his circadian clock and sleep pressure. In this book I share sample schedules with possible sleep and feeding times (see page 79), but you might find that another schedule works better for you, your baby, and your family. That's perfectly fine. Do whatever works best for you—just keep doing it at the same times every day, and your baby will get on a schedule.

> As baby grows, he will feed less frequently and therefore be able to sleep longer at night, and his total twenty-four-hour sleep need will decrease.

The power of How Babies Sleep is that thanks to your fairly strict schedule, which promotes a strong rhythm, your baby will counterintuitively be more flexible with changes in her environment and her routine. She will learn when it is time to eat, when it is time to sleep, and when it is time to play. If something in her schedule changes one day—for example, you put her down later one night because you stayed out—she will be okay with that. Baby will know that she is cranky because it's bedtime, and not cry inconsolably due to a vague feeling of discontent. You can even explain to her that she is tired and will go to sleep soon. She'll be much easier to calm down, because she knows it's true—after all, this is what happens every single day.

> The power of How Babies Sleep is that thanks to your fairly strict schedule, which promotes a strong rhythm, your baby will counterintuitively be more flexible with changes in her environment and her routine.

On a physiological level, a strong rhythm organizes baby's bodily functions and behaviors in an efficient way by anticipating regularly occurring events. Your baby will anticipate wake-up time, feeding time, playtime, bedtime, and so on not just mentally but physically. He doesn't have to work so hard to react to his environment, because his rhythm and his clock are already prepared for what's next. This inner structure allows space for ad hoc changes in baby's schedule, whether it's an early lunch, a new babysitter, or a different crib because you are traveling. In my sleep coaching experience, establishing a robust rhythm has a strong organizing and calming effect not only on baby's body, but also on his psyche, allowing him to be more adaptable and meet changes with relative equanimity.

CREATE THE IDEAL SLEEP AND NAP SCHEDULE
Key Points

★ Establish a sleep schedule for baby based on your ideal bed and wake times.

★ Make sure baby doesn't nap too much during the day, so that he can sleep better at night.

★ Routines entrain baby's rhythm and make transitions easier.

★ As your baby grows, she will need less sleep; adjust the sleep schedule periodically to keep up with her growth and new sleep need.

Step 3: Teach Your Baby to Sleep through the Night

Now we have learned about the power of the clock and how blue morning light entrains it while waking you up and suppressing melatonin. You know to use red light during Night Mode until it's time to wake, and that you, the parent, get to set that time. You also learned about total daily sleep and how naps are inversely correlated with nighttime sleep, translating into a simple rule: don't let baby nap too long, and follow the baby sleep chart (page 30) to determine how much to let baby sleep during the day and when to put her down at night.

Now that you have all of these basics down, we're ready to tackle the final frontier: sleep training to help baby sleep through the night without night feeds and without nighttime crying.

Chapter 12

Signs of Readiness

When baby is about three to four months old or weighs eleven pounds and sometimes sleeps longer stretches (six hours or more) at night, you can start sleep training. This means you will drop night feeds until baby either sleeps through the night for six to eight hours, or, if she wakes up and cries, is able to soothe herself and go back to sleep without parental assistance or feeding. Apart from age, you can look for the following *signs of readiness*.

Baby weighs more than eleven pounds
Babies as young as two months old are able to sleep more than five hours at night, as researchers led by Barbara Galland from New Zealand have found. This sleep duration correlates with a weight of around eleven pounds. Heraghty and colleagues showed in 2008 that preterm babies and babies born with a low birth weight need longer to develop mature sleep patterns. Most doctors and researchers say that babies are generally physically capable of sleeping more than five hours in a stretch at night when they hit the eleven-pound mark.

Baby's night sleep is erratic
If baby's first sleep stretch at night varies vastly from night to night, say three hours one night and six hours another, your baby is

showing you that he doesn't *need* to eat every three hours anymore. It doesn't mean he doesn't want to!

Baby has slept for a longer stretch

If baby has slept even once for a longer stretch at night, say six hours, she has proven to you that she in fact can go for that long without food. Remind yourself of that when sleep training at night.

Baby doesn't seem hungry

If baby cries for you but then quickly loses interest in eating, that's a sign he's not that hungry, and is eating for comfort rather than hunger. If you are breastfeeding, he might not want the second breast, and if you're bottle feeding, he might not finish his bottle.

HOW BABIES SLEEP SUCCESS STORY:
Signs of Readiness for Gentle Sleep Training

I'd been working with Skye and her baby, Henry, since he was twelve weeks old. At three months, baby Henry showed all the signs of sleep readiness: He had slept for more than six hours at night (once as long as seven hours). He weighed thirteen pounds. And when Skye nursed him overnight less than six hours after the last feed, he didn't seem to be hungry, and appeared to be nursing just for comfort.

It was time to start Gentle Sleep Training. I advised Skye to not nurse Henry until five hours after his bedtime feeding, no matter when he woke up. Why five hours? I recommended starting with a no-feed duration of one hour less than the longest the baby has slept on at least two separate occasions; in this case, six hours less one, or five hours.

Then I told Skye to wait ninety seconds before entering Henry's room when he started crying. In order to not be tempted to nurse him, I suggested having her husband placate Henry if he woke before the next feeding time, so Henry didn't anticipate milk. Sleep training can be hard in the early days, so it's also helpful to take turns. If done with discipline, for babies Henry's age, Gentle Sleep Training works almost instantly and can be over after one or two nights. This was the case with Henry, and after just two nights everybody was happily sleeping through the night.

Even if your baby has not demonstrated the ability to sleep longer stretches at night, the vast majority of babies are physically capable of sleeping for at least six hours overnight by around four months of age. By this age, baby may want the comfort of a bottle or breastfeeding or even being held by mom or dad, but he doesn't *need* the food or comfort. Know that!

Once you see these signs of readiness or baby reaches four months of age, you can start sleep training. This is admittedly the hardest part of my entire program, but I am making it as gentle as possible. It will only take a few nights. Keep in mind that *your baby is fine* even if he or she cries for a few minutes.

Chapter 13

Gentle Sleep Training

Here is my simple four-step program:

Step 1. Adjust naps as necessary. Consult the baby sleep chart on page 30 to determine if your baby is sleeping more often or for longer than other babies his age. If so, follow the guidelines in chapter 10 to gently keep baby awake more during the day. Even if the total daytime sleep seems age appropriate, you may still want to slightly reduce daytime napping. Doing so will make baby more tired at night, strongly reducing the crying during sleep training.

Step 2. Follow your bedtime routine and timing. Start Night Mode, turn on the red light, and feed baby thirty minutes before putting her down. Tell her it's now time to sleep.

Step 3. Make a pact with yourself and make a plan. How many hours are you going to wait before feeding baby? How long will you let baby cry? Set a no-feed period that is one hour less than your baby's longest sleep stretch. Remember, you want this to be a reasonable goal, because delaying night feeds isn't easy! Placate your baby without nursing, and ideally without picking him up. Nursing mothers should enlist their partner's (or a family member's) help during night wakings. Your baby won't expect to nurse from your husband or partner. If your partner resists, assure him it will be over in a few nights. Remember, parents have a heightened neurological responsiveness to baby, as explained in the introduction and in chapter 18, so doing this together will help you both get through the stress of sleep training.

Step 4. Let your baby cry for at least ninety seconds. Studies show that waiting one minute to ninety seconds before comforting your baby makes a big difference on the path to sleeping through the night. Even though it's not long, it teaches baby to self-soothe (see page 56). If you can wait a little longer, like two or even five minutes, that's even better. Sometimes baby isn't all-out crying, but is just fussing a bit. If that's the case, try to wait it out. Then, when your baby is crying, send your partner in to placate the baby, but only for one to two minutes. He can shush and pat baby to let her know she's not alone and that parents are aware of her distress and are there. Then he needs to leave the room. Come back after another ninety seconds (or longer). Repeat. Usually it takes three to four cycles: wait—go in—tummy rub and shush for one to two minutes—leave before baby goes back to sleep. This takes about forty-five minutes total before baby goes back to sleep, potentially longer the first two nights you're doing it. If she wakes up and cries again before the no-feed limit is up, repeat the steps above until she's asleep again. (See my "Gentle Sleep Training" illustration on page 116.)

If baby goes back to sleep and sleeps through your no-feed period—perfect! Happy sleeping! Your baby just learned that he can calm himself, and by repeating this he will learn quickly to sleep through the night without your help. When he wakes up next time, and it's past your no-feed limit, wait the ninety seconds as before, but then it's okay to feed him. He held up really well and now it's time for a scheduled feed.

After this first nighttime feed—whether scheduled or unplanned—her second sleep will be shorter. Again, set yourself a no-feed period for another three or four hours after the first feed—however long feels comfortable to you—and follow the same pattern as before—waiting, then soothing without picking up, then waiting, then soothing without picking up.

These first nights of sleep training are hard. You're exhausted and it's very upsetting to hear your baby cry like that. Use your partner as much as possible, and set yourself clear time limits, as in: "I'll wait ninety seconds before going in," using a watch or our Kulala baby sleep app (see page 193 and the last page) to track your progress. Even if you do all this, you might still need to give in and nurse or feed baby before your no-feed period is over. That's okay, as long as you wait at least a few hours after bedtime before nursing or feeding baby, and as long as you let him cry for at least a minute and a half before rushing in. As you continue to sleep train, you can extend the no-feed period, and it will get easier.

I understand that babies' cries are heartbreaking. Babies don't have a sense of time yet, and when they feel uncomfortable, they want you immediately. Why do they feel uncomfortable in the first place, given that they have eaten and are wearing a fresh diaper? Why do babies cry so much? The short answer: we're not entirely sure. Babies' minds are immature, and psychologists believe that they can feel whole only through us, their parents and caregivers, who respond to their needs. The big question is, can we do that—respond to their needs—while also taking care of ourselves by teaching them to sleep through the night? My answer is a resounding yes. This Gentle Sleep Training method teaches them that they will be fine even if they cry for a few minutes, that you're there for them, and that it's okay to sleep now and go for a little longer before the next feed.

HOW BABIES SLEEP SUCCESS STORY:
Gentle Sleep Training

Maria and her partner were nearing exhaustion because their four-month-old baby, James, barely slept at night. He was still sleeping in his parents' room and he was very hard to put down, and needed to be carried around to fall asleep in his parents' arms. Once asleep, he woke up every few hours, some nights even as frequently as every twenty minutes. Furthermore, James liked to have an inopportune "playtime" between 3 and 5 a.m. His parents were at their wits' end.

I coached Maria on how to put the How Babies Sleep method into practice. Even though James was four months old, his sleep total lined up with a typical six-month-old's: he napped for two and a half hours during the day and slept ten hours overnight. The problem was that Maria was putting him down at 7 p.m. for a 7 a.m. wake-up time, which was too early: that's why he was getting up for two hours overnight. We set a wake time of 8 a.m., and created a new bedtime of 9:30 p.m. As this was much later than his original 7 p.m. bedtime, it would be hard to keep him awake till then. So I recommended stretching the time between his naps so that he had his last nap in the early evening to carry him over to this new bedtime. Also, his bedtime routine—bath, book, song, nursing or feeding—could be drawn out at first and start as early as 8:30 p.m. This way the parents and James had structured activities that transitioned him to his new bedtime.

James was also showing all the signs of sleep training readiness: He once slept almost five hours overnight. He didn't seem hungry during night feedings. And he weighed more than eleven pounds. I counseled Maria on how to set a no-feed time (three or four hours) and then wait ninety seconds before soothing James, and enlisting her partner's help.

After just five days, the How Babies Sleep method worked wonders for James and his parents. Maria reported, "Everything is much better with James after our talk. We followed your guidance for the Gentle Sleep Training and made some other adjustments according to your advice. Now his largest sleep is always at least three hours, and we even got a six-hour(!) chunk one night and five hours another—both of which are longer than he's ever slept before without waking. He's generally going down much easier and self-soothing sometimes too. You were right—he can do it!"

This hardest part of sleep training will be over after only two to three nights, after which you can expect a jagged curve, night after night, where baby will wake up at various times (see "The Jagged Curve to Nighttime Sleep" illustration on page 119). Stick with it, and she'll be sleeping longer week by week, even though day by day there will be setbacks.

Although sleep training can be hard, it's important to be consistent. Don't feed your baby when you go in before the no-feed time is up. If you're breastfeeding, know that babies are strongly attracted to and soothed by mother's milk, so much so that just the smell of milk calms down preemies in the ICU during unpleasant procedures. If you go in to placate baby during the no-feed period and baby won't soothe without nursing or feeding, send your husband or partner in to comfort the baby. After a week or two, you'll feel comfortable stretching the first no-feeding period to 4 a.m., then to

5, 6, and eventually 7 a.m. and your desired wake time. Your baby may keep waking up and crying during the night, and you or your partner will keep comforting him without feeding. Before too long, he will learn to be able to go back to sleep without food.

One by one, you'll drop all subsequent night feeds, until only one feed is left, which eventually merges with his wake-up feed.

An example schedule for sleep training for a three-month-old could look like this:

THREE-MONTH-OLD BABY

8:30 a.m.—start of Day Mode	Wake and feed
10:30 a.m.	Nap
11:30 a.m.	Wake
12:00 p.m.	Feed
2:00 p.m.	Nap
4:00 p.m.	Wake and feed
6:15 p.m.	Nap
7:00 p.m.	Wake and feed
9:15 p.m.	Start bedtime routine
9:30 p.m.	Bath
9:45 p.m.—start of Night Mode	Feed and sleep
2:00 a.m.	Feed and sleep
6:00 a.m.	Feed and sleep

If baby wakes up during the no-feed zones between 10 p.m. and 2 a.m. or 2 a.m. and 6 a.m., use Gentle Sleep Training to soothe baby without feeding until it's time to feed again. Increase the no-feed zone from four to five hours, and eventually six, then seven hours.

For other ages, consult baby sleep schedules on page 79, or use the Kulala baby sleep app to create your custom schedule (see page 193 and the last page).

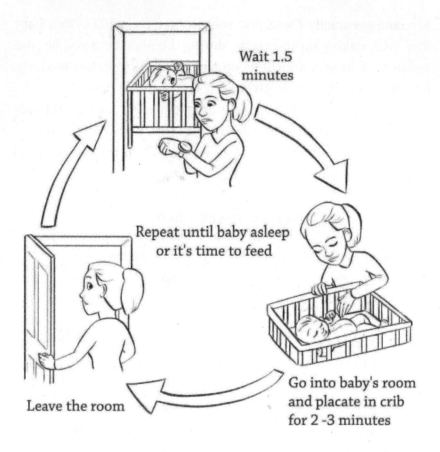

Wait 1.5 minutes

Repeat until baby asleep or it's time to feed

Leave the room

Go into baby's room and placate in crib for 2 -3 minutes

Gentle Sleep Training
When baby starts crying during the night, wait for at least ninety seconds. Look at your watch and take a deep breath. You're not harming baby if you let her cry for a minute and a half. Go in and soothe her, and then leave the room after two to three minutes, even if she is still crying or starts crying as soon as you leave. Repeat.

Sleeping through the night

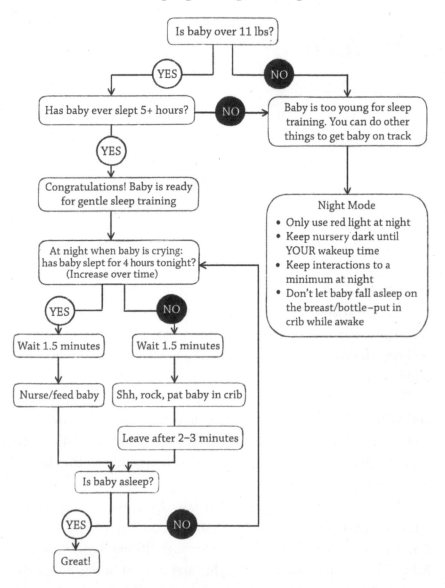

Is your baby ready for sleep training? Use this flowchart to check for the important signs.

Chapter 14

Is It Working?

Sleep training is hard, because baby will cry inconsolably, and you will feel guilty for depriving her of food. What if she really needs to eat? If your baby ever sleeps for longer stretches, you can rest assured: she does not need to eat. Stay strong—you know that to establish a good sleep pattern you must reinforce the desired rhythm. If you give in, you not only weaken the "good" rhythm, you actually set baby off on a wrong rhythm, making her think the middle of the night is a proper feeding time.

This method is highly effective, so if you try this for a week and your baby still wakes up predictably after only a few hours of nighttime sleep, reexamine his daytime sleep (refer to the baby sleep chart on page 30). If he sleeps too many hours during the day, he won't sleep as well at night.

Most parents I work with want to know: *How long will it take until my baby sleeps through the night?* First, what do we mean by sleeping through the night? I define sleeping through the night as when your baby's longest sleep stretch at night lasts at least seven hours. So when will this important milestone be reached? With Gentle Sleep Training, you will see a trend of baby sleeping longer stretches at night. The curve will not be smooth, but jagged (see "The Jagged Curve to Nighttime Sleep" illustration on page 119). What I mean by this is that if you look at baby's general sleep schedule over a month, you'll see that her overnight sleep stretch is lengthening, but day to day it will vary, and your baby will likely keep waking up at different times during the night.

Don't get discouraged when a spell of longer sleeping is terminated by a week of regression with shorter bouts of sleep. Your

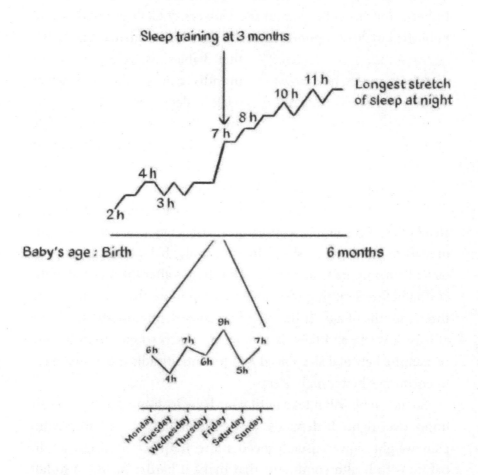

The Jagged Curve to Nighttime Sleep
Over the course of weeks and months, baby's longest stretch of nighttime sleep increases (top), but from day to day there is high variability (bottom). After sleep training, which is usually possible starting at around three months, baby will sleep much longer at night. With my program, most sleep-trained babies can sleep eleven hours at night by six months of age.

sleep training is working, but it takes time. Don't stop everything you are doing. Keep your daytime schedule, keep the shortened daytime naps, keep bedtime and wake time and all routines. Don't lose faith—baby will sleep through the night if you stick with the program, because How Babies Sleep is based on baby's biology.

Moreover, research conducted by lead author Ian St James-Roberts and his colleagues at the University College London and published in 2017 supports my method. Video evidence has shown that babies as young as three months can soothe themselves back to sleep rather quickly without parental intervention. How soon it happens depends on that little delay we introduce, those one and a half minutes we allow baby to learn self-soothing, instead of creating an unnecessary sleep association of needing mom or dad to fall back to sleep. In this study, babies whose parents waited one minute to one and a half minutes after the onset of night crying before soothing were able to sleep more than five hours by three months of age. If the schedule consistently doesn't work for at least a week, and baby is waking up much sooner than before, reexamine her total sleep need and potentially adjust daytime naps to encourage better night sleep.

> Video evidence has shown that babies as young as three months can soothe themselves back to sleep rather quickly without parental intervention.

So how long will it take until your baby is sleeping at least seven hours overnight? It depends. Some factors are clear: babies who gain weight slower usually need more frequent feedings, as do babies with health conditions that make it harder for them to fall asleep. The most important factor, however, is your perseverance. Hearing baby cry takes an emotional toll on parents, especially mothers, as described in the introduction and in chapter 18. That's why enlisting a partner's help can be crucial. Using my method, most babies will consistently sleep for at least one six-hour stretch

HOW BABIES SLEEP SUCCESS STORY:
Sleeping through the Night

Amelia was three months old and showing signs of readiness for sleep training. I had already worked with her mom, Julie, to address her light exposure, reduce her naps, and move bedtime later. But Amelia was still waking up during the night. Amelia weighed more than eleven pounds, and had slept more than eight hours at night a few times, so she was ready for Gentle Sleep Training. I explained the basics to Julie, including why waiting just ninety seconds can help babies sleep through the night faster than babies who are immediately soothed. After the first sleep coaching session, Amelia slept like a dream. It took only three nights to wean her off night feeds, and she was now sleeping in nine-to-ten-hour stretches at night.

during the night by four months of age, and sleep through the night in a seven-hour stretch between four and five months.

Tweaking Baby's Schedule

Once the schedule has been set and sleep training is working, you will start to feel like a new person. Your baby will eat and sleep at predictable times, which will make his and your life much easier. He will sleep during most of the night, and you'll be back to your old self. Even if he feeds frequently at night, he understands that night is for sleeping, which means your nighttime feeding sessions will be quick and painless, and you can all go back to sleep right after. Congratulate yourself, because the hardest part of sleep training is done! Mission accomplished!

From here on, you will only need to periodically tweak the schedule as your baby grows and her sleep and food needs change. As baby gets older, she might be able to go longer without milk. This will be a gradual process and you might slowly increase the interval between feeds from two to three and a half or even four hours during the day. Around the six-month mark (or sometimes earlier) most parents introduce solid food, which adds another element to the baby's schedule. Refer to the table on page 79 for examples of feeding and nap schedules for different ages.

Chapter 15

Sleep Regressions

There's a very common pattern that I see in my coaching practice. After I've worked with a family and helped them effectively sleep train, everybody is happy. Baby sleeps at night, and so do parents. A few months pass, and suddenly I get another email like this one:

> "We don't know what happened, but Miles suddenly stopped sleeping well at night. He now wakes up every hour and screams bloody murder. I have to nurse him to calm him down, or my husband has to carry him around for hours before he stops crying. Help!"

Usually the parents have a culprit for why their baby stopped sleeping well at night.

> "We were in London for a week and now his sleep is all messed up."

> "He started daycare."

> "She's teething, so I think she is in pain and can't sleep well."

> "I went back to work last week—I think she is unsettled by this change."

While these are all valid concerns, they are largely—with the exception of jet lag—irrelevant to baby's sleep. In 90 percent of cases there is a single reason why baby has suddenly stopped sleeping so well. Can you guess what it is? It's too much napping.

> In 90 percent of cases there is a single reason why baby has suddenly stopped sleeping so well. . . . Too much napping.

We learned in step 2 that babies' total sleep continuously decreases from birth, when they sleep, well, most of the time, to adulthood, when it's just around eight hours a night. In the first two years of life, your baby's total sleep need decreases dramatically, from sixteen hours a day to around twelve. If you want your baby to keep sleeping eleven to twelve hours at night, where is most of the sleep lost, then? That's right—during the day.

While nighttime sleep doesn't change much between six months and five years, daytime sleep undergoes big changes. Babies go from napping eight hours during the day as newborns to completely dropping naps when they are three or four years old. What's confusing for parents is that babies are going to keep their total daily sleep constant no matter what—they don't care whether they sleep during the day or during the night—and they don't always give clear signs that they need to drop or shorten their nap. Instead they will just fight bedtime, wake up in the middle of the night, or get up too early. If parents let them sleep too much during the day, their nighttime sleep will be reduced—and, conversely, if daytime naps are shorter, nighttime sleep is increased. So it's really up to you: Can you keep baby awake during the day, standing the occasional crankiness during the transition period, for the benefit of sleeping at night? Or do you prefer a napping baby during the day—at the expense of sleeping through the night? Most parents prioritize night sleep!

Just as with the families I coached, at some point after your schedule is established, with baby eating and napping on the clock and blissfully sleeping through the night, there will be trouble in paradise. Suddenly baby will wake up in the middle of the night and it will be hard to put her back to sleep. Or bedtime will become a drawn-out struggle. When it happens once or twice, you will think it's a fluke. However, after it has been going on almost every day for a week, you realize something is off. *What is happening?* Most likely, your baby has grown and her daily sleep need has decreased. The solution is easy. Reduce daytime sleep—baby needs to nap less.

To determine how much time you need to skim off naps, compare your baby's sleep schedule to the chart on page 30—and use our Kulala baby sleep app (see page 193 and the last page). Let's say that before this sleep regression, your baby needed fifteen hours of sleep every day, but now it's only fourteen hours. In order to keep her nighttime sleep consistent, you have to reduce her total daytime napping by one hour. Otherwise, she will wake in the middle of the night, fight bedtime, or wake very early in the morning—none of which is good for mom and dad. It may take a few days of trial and error before you cut the right amount from her naps and see the desired result: baby sleeps through the night again.

HOW BABIES SLEEP SUCCESS STORY:
Sleep Regression

I first helped baby William and his parents, Johanna and David, when he was fourteen weeks old. Using the How Babies Sleep program, Johanna and David got William to sleep through the night. All was well until the family took a trip to London when William was almost five months old. When they got back, things started to deteriorate. Both nighttime and daytime sleep were a struggle, he was crying to go down for his four daily naps, and he was fighting his last nap. Some days he could not be put down for the afternoon nap at all. He also regressed to waking up multiple times during the night, and it was tough to soothe him back to sleep. By the time Johanna emailed me for help, they were both exhausted.

Johanna and David felt like the jet lag was to blame for William's sleep problems. They were partly right—it takes up to a week to adjust to a new time zone, especially London to NYC, which are five hours apart. But then he never got back on track after readjusting to New York time. That's because William was three and a half months old when we established a new sleep schedule, which worked wonderfully for a while. Now, at five months, William didn't need to sleep as much, and we needed to reduce his naps. Between three months and six months of age, babies go from napping an average of four hours a day to only two and a half hours a day. And nighttime sleep increases from ten hours to eleven hours. This means we needed to cut William's naps and make his bedtime earlier. William himself was showing us that he didn't need to sleep as much, because he now sometimes skipped his last nap. That's a sure sign of reduced sleep need. So what to do?

Johanna and David gently reduced each nap to fifty minutes, and dropped the fourth nap altogether. This shift immediately helped with nighttime sleep. What about the nighttime wakings? Back to basics! Johanna and David returned to Gentle Sleep Training. After just two days on his new schedule, William was back to sleeping through the night.

Dropping Naps

"Sometimes he naps, sometimes he doesn't." Sound familiar? If it has been getting harder and harder to put baby down for a particular nap, or if she sometimes skips it altogether, it's time to drop it. Her total sleep need has decreased. Her sleep pressure is lower and therefore she is not as tired. Dropping naps has a bad reputation for being very difficult and resulting in inconsolable babies. It's true that dropping the nap can result in some initial crankiness; however, if it's done right, this will only last for a day or two.

This means that you need to create a new schedule for your baby. Turn to page 79 for sample schedules for different age groups. If you'd prefer to create your own schedule, think about dropping the latest nap, increasing the duration of each nap, and spacing the remaining naps farther apart. You'll also put your baby to sleep earlier, since nighttime sleep increases between one and eighteen months from nine hours to eleven and a half hours. Over the first year and a half of your baby's life, you will transition from four naps a day for a newborn, to three naps from ages three to six months, to two naps from ages six to twelve months, and then one nap until age three or four. The last nap to stay is the one in the afternoon, typically after lunch.

Some crankiness is normal during the transition, but your baby should adjust quite quickly. If she stays very cranky and sleepy for more than three days during her usual nap time, it's probably too early to drop that particular nap.

Another problem situation to watch out for is when bedtime and the last nap become too close together. Because dropping the fourth or later third nap before bedtime is a particularly tricky one, I'd like to delve deeper into how to do it as painlessly as possible. Say your baby has her last nap at 7:30 p.m., and it usually lasts for an hour. Recently she has been sleeping longer and longer at night, and you have been putting her down earlier and earlier, so that now her bedtime is 9 p.m. At this point, when she wakes up at 8:30 p.m., she only has half an hour before it is bedtime proper. The last nap is starting to merge with her nighttime sleep—it's time to drop it! Be prepared to have a fussy baby the first day when you don't put her down for her nap. You can try sticking to her usual bedtime, or put her down up to thirty minutes earlier. The next day she will already be much better, and you just need another day or two for her to fully transition.

If baby remains tired and cranky during the time of the dropped nap for the next three to five days, try moving bedtime even earlier. As long as she sleeps through the night, that is the right thing to do. If she starts waking up at ungodly hours again, you know you went too far, and that her bedtime should be later.

Chapter 16

Sleep Increase

While the general trend is that babies, toddlers, and older kids sleep less and less as they get older (as shown in the baby sleep chart on page 30), there will be phases and times when their sleep increases.

Sickness

Sick babies, children, and adults often have an increased sleep need. It is important to let kids sleep as long as they need to when they are sick. Feverish babies and toddlers especially tend to sleep a lot more during the day than usual. Let them sleep! But what about night sleep, you might wonder. Many parents report that when their kid is sick, their sleep schedule falls apart and they spend the night awake with their screaming baby or toddler. This is where you will particularly reap the benefits of How Babies Sleep—the constant repetition, regular schedule, and keeping strict Night Mode will allow your baby to stay on track. When kids are sick, their overall daily sleep need is higher, but with How Babies Sleep, the increased daytime sleep is unlikely to reduce nighttime sleep. That's the power of entrainment to a strong rhythm! Time and time again when my kids were sick, they were cranky or sleepy during the day, but their nighttime sleep was barely affected. Of course, sometimes sick children wake up during the night and feel miserable and need extra comfort or help.

Naturally, when babies get a little older, they turn into toddlers and can express their suffering and their needs (and you will find they have strong opinions!). There will inevitably be times when you find yourself holding your sick child for hours at night, sleeping with him, and doing whatever you can to help him feel better. Mommy's and daddy's love and affection are very important to help a sick child get better, but they can also form new habits that are hard to break, especially with older children. Therefore, when your baby or toddler starts feeling better, it's imperative to return to normal sleep schedules and routines as soon as possible.

Around two years of age, Leah had a terrible fever, and she refused to sleep without me. She would fall asleep on top of me on the couch in her room. She also woke up multiple times at night, burning up with fever and crying. Each time, she needed me to hold her to go back to sleep. She was sick and miserable, so of course I did everything I could to make her feel better, including staying with her for hours in her room, holding and stroking her. After three days she was feeling better but still wanted me as a nice warm cushion to sleep on. So even after I put her down for the evening, she still called me back multiple times. At first, I thought she might still be feeling ill. But by day four, I realized that we had inadvertently transitioned into a new habit.

On day five, when I was confident she was her playful and energetic self again and didn't feel sick anymore, it was time to return to our regular routine: bath, book, and final cuddle at 9 p.m. and not a sound until 8 a.m. When she called me back after I put her down, I waited before returning, barely able to stand her excruciating crying. I broke down and went back in, giving her a hug but telling her it was time to sleep and Mommy won't come in anymore before it's time to get up. I left. Mad crying again. I broke down again after ten minutes. This continued for another half hour, until I decided to wait longer. She screamed bloody murder for half an hour, but also came up with many creative reasons why I should come and get her (*I need to go potty, I want to play in the living room, I'm hungry*), which showed me she didn't really *need* me, she just wanted me. After what felt like an eternity of crying (but was actually only thirty minutes), I went in and gave her one last hug. She stopped after that and finally went to sleep, this time for the night. The next night she went to sleep after our regular routine without me having to come back and lie with her again and again. The habit was broken, and we were back to our regular routine. Everybody was sleeping happily at night again.

During episodes of sickness, comforting your child takes prece-

 HOW BABIES SLEEP SUCCESS STORY:
Sickness

I coached Oliver's parents when he was five months, and we got him on a great schedule. But when he was nine months old, things suddenly changed. Oliver caught a bad cold and had a high fever for a few days. During his sickness he was crying a lot and needed to be held, calmed down, and nursed frequently. After he felt fine again, his sleep stayed fragmented, and he was waking up four to six times every night, bringing his parents to the brink of exhaustion. His mom, Vanessa, reached out to me for help, and I explained that the extra snuggling and nursing during Oliver's cold had created new, unwelcome habits. She needed to return to Gentle Sleep Training to get back on track. While it was hard for Vanessa to sleep train again for a few nights, the effort paid off: Oliver remembered his self-soothing skills and stopped relying on his parents for sleeping through the night.

dence over all schedules and routines. Babies and toddlers usually need more sleep, more holding, more caressing, and more mom when they are sick. Give them everything they need, but when they feel better, be mindful of not forming a new habit that you will need to break again. It's best to return to your normal pre-sickness schedule as soon as possible. Explain to your baby or toddler that now that she feels better, she can go to sleep alone again, night is for sleeping, and her mommy or daddy will be there in the morning.

Toddler Sleep Increase

Around two years of age, toddlers reach a plateau in their daily sleep need. For the next year their sleep at night is unlikely to go down further, and there might even be monthlong phases where they need significantly more sleep than before (up to an hour is not unusual). This often coincides with starting or progressing in the highly stimulating setting of nursery school, as well as a unique phase of emotional and intellectual development. Rather than having to wake up your child in order to get to school, you can follow How Babies Sleep to rearrange your toddler's schedule so that it works for his changing sleep needs.

> Put him down earlier at night, gradually shifting his bedtime in fifteen-minute increments until the sleep equilibrium is reached again.

Put him down earlier at night, gradually shifting his bedtime in fifteen-minute increments until the sleep equilibrium is reached again and your designated wake time coincides with toddler's filled sleep need. Easy! How Babies Sleep is a constant process of adjusting and readjusting the schedule in place so that the child's nighttime sleep and morning wake time are aligned with yours.

Chapter 17

Other Caregivers

So now you have the basics of this program down pat, and are convinced about using the red light and limiting daytime sleep—but other people in your or baby's life might not be! They might not know that normal light wakes babies up, and that too much napping is detrimental to nighttime sleep. Does it matter if they don't follow the rules from this book? If those people will be taking care of your child, then yes, it does. It matters for two major reasons. We learned that everything we do or don't do either entrains or weakens baby's rhythm, and that a strong rhythm helps her be happier and sleep better. If your partner, the nanny, or daycare attendants have a different schedule for baby than you do, or don't have a schedule at all, that will upend all the work you've put into getting her on a schedule that works for you and your family. Furthermore, if your finely calibrated nap schedule is ignored, and another caregiver lets baby sleep as long as she wants during the day, this will most likely result in sleepless nights. Therefore, it is crucial that everyone is on the same page.

Nursery School

Starting a school or daycare program is challenging for babies and toddlers because they need to get used to new caregivers, other kids,

a different physical environment, and different routines and schedules. A daycare environment is very stimulating for babies and toddlers, and they learn a lot from interacting with teachers and other
kids. They often experience a higher volume of sensory, intellectual,
and social stimulation there than they do at home and are physically
more active than in the home setting. School is tiring! Many babies
and toddlers are exhausted at night when they first start daycare,
which can be difficult for the parents. Putting kids down earlier
seems like the easiest solution, but be careful not to overshoot.

If baby seems extremely tired, you can try putting him down
fifteen or thirty minutes earlier. However, if he wakes up before his
usual wake time or starts waking up during the night, you know
that his sleep need hasn't increased. Instead of putting your child
down earlier, start the bedtime routine earlier, get him in the bath
earlier, and read an extra book. Kids are more tired after school, yes,
but this fatigue does not necessarily translate to an increased sleep
need; it can instead manifest as increased crankiness and clinginess.
They've been away from you all day and they had to pull it together
without you. They need to let it out, and they want you to prove that
you are there for them.

Naps in Daycare

If your baby was on a specific schedule before starting daycare, try
to instruct the new caregivers to keep everything constant. However, waking babies or toddlers up from naps might be met with
resistance due to people's lack of understanding of the biology of
sleep. It may also be challenging for daycare providers to accommo-
date a separate schedule for each child, like if other kids are napping
more (or less) than your little one.

But of course you know that excessive daytime sleep can wreak
havoc on baby's nighttime sleep. Endless napping in daycare will

lead to late bedtimes and sleepless nights. You can explain that you have been waking baby up routinely to restrict daytime sleep and allow for better nighttime sleep, and that this is an accepted method to enable good nighttime sleep. You can describe how this approach has helped your

> Endless napping in daycare will lead to late bedtimes and sleepless nights.

family regain normal sleep at night and how important that is for you. Try to explain your approach to the caregivers, and ideally find out when interviewing nursery schools and daycares if they will cooperate with you on your How Babies Sleep approach.

Keeping the House on a Schedule

It is crucial to be on the same page with everyone in the household about your baby's sleep and feeding schedules. In order to keep to the plan, it is helpful to have an up-to-date schedule on the fridge or in another visible place, so everyone can easily reference feeding and nap times. You've put a lot of valuable time and effort into learning about the science of sleep and have worked hard to get baby on a schedule. Make your partner read this book. Explain your approach and especially why you're limiting daytime sleep to every caregiver. Insist on the importance of your schedule and restricting nap durations. You will likely experience resistance, but it is important to stay firm for baby to keep sleeping well at night.

Chapter 18

Understanding Mom—and Dad— Brain

Sleep training—even the gentle variety I recommend—is by far the hardest part of my method. It's not just you; every mom and dad has a very hard time letting their baby cry. I was no exception. When I was sleep training Leah and Noah, it was almost physically impossible for me to sit still and wait for even ninety seconds—it felt like I was doing serious harm to my baby, and to myself.

Why is it that we're so deeply affected by our baby's cries? Hearing other people cry doesn't usually make us feel that bad, so why are we reacting to baby's crying in such an extreme way? Understanding why we have this strong reaction can help us modulate our panic response—and allow us to proceed with sleep training. This section will help you understand the biology behind the mix of emotions you experience as a parent, and how we can tweak them to help baby sleep through the night.

That surge of love you feel when you look at your baby? Those feelings you never thought were possible? Yeah, that's hormonal. Nature made it so we are not just optimally prepared for baby's arrival on a physical level, with milk production and whatnot, but also on a mental level. Hormones make us love our babies, a lot—to the point where their well-being becomes paramount, even more important than ours. I'm a neuroscientist, so a book about baby sleep would not be complete without taking into consideration how pregnancy, childbirth, and childcare change us, physically and emotionally, and how those changes influence our ability to help baby—and ultimately ourselves—sleep at night.

Hormones during Pregnancy

Before I was pregnant with Leah, my weight and appearance preoccupied a not too small part of my waking existence, and keeping in shape was important to me. Fluctuations in my weight did, maybe disproportionally, affect my mood. When I became pregnant, and my belly started to grow, this fragile—and demanding—relationship with my body profoundly changed. After the months of feeling sick all the time, when my belly started to show I was strangely happy about it. And then when it became bigger, I was in awe, and could not believe that it was to become yet bigger, and bigger, and bigger. Toward the end, I was feeling uncomfortable, sure, but my appearance, my almost grotesquely changed body—speaking from the perspective of my self-critical pre-pregnant self—didn't bother me too much, or at least not as much as you would expect for someone for whom five pounds more or less had been life-changing in the years before. When I was actually able to put the dinner plate on my belly while watching TV, this manifestation of enormity elicited only mild amusement.

Apart from my lack of body dysmorphia over my Kafkaesque transformation into a house, I also experienced a general lack of worry given that something outrageous was happening to my body and my life, and everything was about to change in the most unimaginable, existential way. Yes, of course I was worried—about the baby being healthy, about giving birth, about being a good mom. But my fears and worries were somehow relatively small in relation to the actual significance of the things that were about to happen. Even while I was pregnant, I commented to my friends and family on the strangeness of not experiencing pregnancy as very stressful—how changing in this absurd way would have freaked me out enormously before, but that I was oddly calm about everything now that I was actually doing it. Most mothers report such a sense of relative calm, and they almost feel like they are destined to go through this experience.

Science can provide an amazing explanation for this phenomenon. Exposure to stress, which causes elevated levels of the hormone cortisol in the mother, can harm the developing fetus. Nature came up with a system to prevent that. During pregnancy, a complicated interplay of brain chemistry and hormones modulates the so-called hypothalamic-pituitary-adrenal (HPA) axis—a physiological chain of events involving the hypothalamus in the brain hormonally signaling to the pituitary gland, which in turn controls the adrenal gland, located above the kidneys, to release cortisol. This whole process is dampened during pregnancy and held in check through the action of the hormone progesterone and endogenous opioids, which peak in late pregnancy and suppress the HPA axis, reducing stress when you're pregnant.

What's particularly fascinating is that even partners of pregnant women show hormonal changes during pregnancy. Male testosterone declines during a partner's pregnancy, and this is necessary for father-infant bonding after the baby is born. Furthermore, couples' hormones change in sync, preparing the parental unit for optimal childcare.

Hormones during Childbirth

You've probably heard of the "cuddle hormone" oxytocin, which produces such astounding prosocial effects as increasing someone's perceived attractiveness after it's sprayed into one's nose, increasing trust in others, and even improving "mind reading"—understanding intuitively what others want and need.

Oxytocin's most profound function is in childbirth. During late pregnancy, oxytocin neurons are inhibited through endogenous opioids, but when the baby is ready to come out, this opioid inhibition is released—and oxytocin neurons begin to fire reflexively and release oxytocin, triggering uterine convulsions—labor contractions. Pitocin, the drug used to enhance labor, is a chemical analog of oxytocin, illustrating the powerful role of the hormone in squeezing the baby through the birth canal. Simultaneously with labor, the hormones prolactin and oxytocin trigger lactation. After the baby is born, suckling on mother's breast triggers oxytocin in both mother and baby, which in turn leads to the letdown reflex and milk flow.

Postpartum Hormones

During pregnancy, the maternal brain gets prepared for motherhood, which, biologically speaking, includes nesting, gathering the young, nursing, cleaning, protecting, and staying nonaggressive toward the new baby. Elevated levels of estrogen, progesterone, and prolactin "prime" various parts of the maternal brain by increasing the amount of oxytocin receptors. The brain is ready to go—and when progesterone drops and oxytocin is released during childbirth, these neural pathways start firing, eliciting maternal behaviors.

It is truly astounding to consider the vastness of reorganization happening to the new mother's brain. Virtually all brain areas related to cognitive and emotional processing are altered by the concerted action of pregnancy hormones and respond strongly to the surge of oxytocin during childbirth. In fact, when mice are missing oxytocin receptors (because they have been genetically knocked out), they don't show maternal behaviors after their pups are born. They don't care for their young, and even become aggressive toward them.

Interestingly, prolonged interaction with the newborn is important to sustain and reinforce maternal behaviors postpartum. This is why bonding with the new baby is so important. While our brains are primed for maternal behaviors, it's the contact with the new baby that solidifies the neural pathways for sustained child-rearing and responsiveness to baby's needs. Continuous interaction and care for baby activates powerful reward circuits in our brain, causing the release of the neurotransmitter dopamine, which makes us feel good. Those are the same brain circuits activated by drug use, and the same ones firing when you're in love.

In fact, after my first baby, Leah, was born, I felt such intense love, I considered writing a sonnet. While I didn't actually put pen to paper, due to constant diaper changing and lack of Shakespearean talent, I suddenly understood those centuries of writers and poets experiencing such overwhelming feelings of love that only writing poems would adequately express their inner life. I wanted to pour my heart into poetry, compose symphonies, and create books (well, I did *that* at least) to celebrate the almost spiritual exhilaration I felt—for my baby daughter, her magical existence, and her blue eyes, looking at me, needing me.

Following the newborn phase, we remain intimately connected to baby's cues. Research shows that all three members of the family—mothers, fathers, and infants—experience oxytocin increases upon interaction with each other, which reinforces bonding and parental behaviors. Baby and parents form a functional triad, with synchronized hormones, neural pathways, and behaviors. This is where intuition and secure attachment come from. The baby makes us care for her, and we reciprocally make her feel secure by taking care of her, all the while fine-tuning our behaviors to optimally tend to her—all these steps are biologically predetermined yet constantly evolving to facilitate one of the most intense and beautiful experiences of humankind: becoming a parent.

As you can imagine, it's not all roses and butterflies. New parents are preoccupied with their babies to the point of self-abandonment, and worry endlessly about baby's well-being. While this is crucial for baby's survival, it can cause high levels of stress in new parents. This experience has a biological explanation, uncovered by a series of interesting experiments.

When new mothers and fathers were shown images of their babies crying, and their brain activity was simultaneously monitored using functional magnetic resonance imaging, the researchers detected strong responses in a brain center called the amygdala, which is something like our emotional panic button. We perceive our baby's cries as unbearable, and we have brain reactions to show it. Parts of our brain that signal emotional alarm light up like a Christmas tree when our baby cries, and that causes us immense distress.

Interestingly, while fathers also respond to their babies' cries, mothers' brain responses are much more pronounced than fathers'. This fits well with many mothers' everyday observation of being fully awakened by baby's slightest noise, while daddy continues to happily snore through any amount of baby's screaming. How can he? He can because his emotional alarm center doesn't go off at baby's every sound. While this extreme physiological and emotional response somewhat subsides after a while—parents of six-month-olds show much weaker amygdala responses than parents of two-week-old babies—the state of heightened emotional responsiveness is of course part of the job description of being a parent, facilitating intense bonding and love but also anxiety and sometimes depression.

Parents' preoccupation with their new baby is so intense and stereotypical, it resembles a set of behaviors typical of obsessive-compulsive disorder. Before you—understandably—feel offended, think about it: anxiously examining and reexamining baby's vitals—check. Constantly worrying you forgot something relating to baby's well-being or even survival—check. Pervasive disturbing and recurring thoughts relating to harm coming to baby—check. The similarities, specifically on a neurological level, are so uncanny, researchers are even using imaging of mothers' brains as a means to understand obsessive-compulsive behavior and its evolutionary origins.

The Function of Sleep

You probably picked up this book because your baby doesn't sleep well and you're not feeling well yourself. Why is that? What is it about sleep that is so vital to our well-being? Why do we need to sleep at all?

These are the very questions I study in my day-to-day job as a sleep scientist, and the short answer is: we're not sure. To be precise, what we are not sure about is the ultimate, underlying, basic function of sleep—what is the number one thing sleep is accomplishing in our bodies, which, when it doesn't happen due to sleep deprivation, makes us miserable and, ultimately, ill?

This question was also intensely studied by Allan Rechtschaffen and colleagues from the University of Chicago. The researchers deprived rats of sleep, using a rotating disk placed above a pool of water. The disk would be bisected by a screen, and one rat would be placed on each side of the screen. As soon as one of the rats— the one destined to be sleep deprived—would fall asleep, the disk would start rotating, but the screen would stay put, threatening to push the rat into the water. To prevent an unwelcome swimming excursion, the rat would have to start moving instead of sleeping. This disk-over-water method allows researchers to investigate what happens during total sleep deprivation, when an animal is not allowed to sleep at all.

Rats subjected to this torturous method died within two weeks—that is sooner than death from food deprivation! Why is total sleep deprivation lethal? After a few days of not sleeping, the rats started showing a plethora of physical and physiological aberrations, including disheveled and clumped fur, lowered body temperature, weight loss, infection, skin ulcers, and brain changes. The weird thing was that no single reason for their death was found: when the researchers helped the rats to feel warmer, gave them antibiotics to control their infection, and took other counter-measures against the effects of sleep deprivation, the rats still died. Why—remains a mystery.

Molecular biologists like myself have continued the search for the function of sleep and discovered a number of physiological processes that occur in our cells and tissues when we sleep. Without going into the technical details of ongoing research, we believe that sleep has something to do with maintenance of basic cellular functions in the brain and the body. On a brain level, we all know how not getting enough sleep impairs our functioning, and while we don't fully understand why, I want to delve a little deeper into the effects of sleep deprivation on the brain.

The Sleep-Deprived Brain

To investigate how sleep deprivation affects humans, researchers have subjected groups of people to varying degrees of sleep deprivation. In one study from the University of Pennsylvania, subjects in one group were not allowed to sleep at all for three consecutive nights, while another group was subjected to partial sleep deprivation and allowed to sleep for either four hours or six hours per night for fourteen days. This and other studies showed that sleep deprivation has profound detrimental effects on brain functions including attention and motivation, working and long-term memory, visual processing, decision making and judgment, speech, and emotional control.

Maybe unsurprisingly, the more sleep deprived you are, the worse the symptoms are. Interestingly, not just total but also partial sleep deprivation—the state new mothers find themselves in—has negative effects on cognition and emotional regulation. Missing two hours of sleep per night for fourteen days is as bad as one night of total sleep deprivation. The consequences? Research shows that groups at risk for habitual sleep deprivation, including workers in medical, aviation, military, or trans-

> Sleep deprivation has profound detrimental effects on brain functions including attention and motivation, working and long-term memory, visual processing, decision making and judgment, speech, and emotional control.

HOW BABIES SLEEP SUCCESS STORY:
Sleep Deprivation

Carla reached out to me when baby Matteo was seven months old. Matteo was a happy, active baby during the day, but at night he was waking up at two-hour intervals, driving his mother crazy. He was taking four naps during the day, totaling five hours. Carla was an engineer but had not been able to return to work at baby Matteo's six-month mark, which put the family under substantial economic strain. "I need to be able to think during my job, but right now I feel like a zombie," she told me. I explained that Matteo was napping too much, and taught Carla the steps of Gentle Sleep Training. After implementing the new schedule and sleep training Matteo, Carla got her sleep back and was able to return to work a month later.

portation fields, display impaired vigilance and are more prone to errors due to sleep deprivation. One study from the University of New South Wales, in Australia, and the New Zealand Occupational and Environmental Health Research Centre indeed found that after twenty-eight hours without sleep, army and transportation personnel were as cognitively impaired as drunk persons with a blood alcohol level of 0.1 percent. While women seem to be more resilient to sleep deprivation than men, probably due to the demands of child rearing, I cannot stress enough how important it is for you to get back to sleeping well—for your sake and for your family's sake.

Sleep and Mood

I have had sleep problems for as long as I can remember. As a child, I had trouble sleeping, and would lie awake in the middle of the night, my thoughts keeping me awake. While medicating me with sleeping pills was out of the question for my parents, at one point they brought in a homeopath to help, a very nice lady who interviewed me for three hours, and then prescribed special "globuli"—tiny sugar balls that contained trace amounts of plant extracts supposedly beneficial for sleep. While I liked the one-on-one attention and concern I received, the globuli did nothing for my sleep. What ended up being somewhat helpful was my father—a psychiatrist—teaching me relaxation techniques, which I sometimes used when I was lying in bed and couldn't fall asleep.

As a young adult, I had erratic sleep schedules, and I didn't know until I joined my current laboratory at Rockefeller University that for insomniacs this lack of structure aggravates sleep problems. In college I could be up at 7 a.m. one day and at 2 p.m. the next, and when I studied for my Diplom (the German equivalent of a master's degree), my whole rhythm flipped and I lived out of phase with society, getting up at 5 p.m. and going to bed when the sun came up. Due to my erratic schedule, I was living a vicious cycle where I'd sleep in only to not be able to fall asleep the next night, wake up sleep deprived, sleep in, and so on. I might feel okay one day and then suffer horribly from lack of sleep the next.

When I am sleep deprived, which for me constitutes getting less than seven hours of sleep, I don't feel well. I'm not just tired; my mood is impacted. I don't have energy or motivation, and I feel depressed. Maybe that's why I was so eager to prevent sleep deprivation when my kids were born—to prevent the perfect storm of poor sleep and feeling depressed.

And I'm not alone in this. There is a strong association between sleep and mood. Poor sleep leads to poor mood, and sleep quality is directly associated with how a new mother feels in the first days, weeks, and months postpartum. Multiple studies have shown that a new mother's poor sleep in the postpartum period increases the risk for developing baby blues—a temporary phase of depressive symptoms, which occurs in up to 85 percent of new mothers. In one study, low mood in mothers of one-week-old babies was entirely explained by mom's nighttime wakefulness—how well she was able to sleep through the night. In 2000 Kathryn Lee and colleagues from the University of California, San Francisco performed polysomnography studies on women before and after delivery to track sleep changes in new mothers and understand how they related to mood. They reported that at one month after delivery, mothers slept on average 1.7 hours less than they had during their third trimester. What's more, that sleep duration one month postpartum tracked with mood: mothers who were in a good mood—called positive affect—slept on average 1.3 more hours than the mothers who were experiencing negative affect—mothers who felt depressed.

In another study, poor sleep at one week postpartum was even predictive of developing an episode of postpartum depression at six weeks postpartum, illustrating how important sleep is for our mental health. In these studies, it is hard to tease apart what comes first—poor sleep or low mood. Does sleep disturbance cause mood disorders, or vice versa? Researchers believe that both are true—and that they can cause a vicious feedback loop: sleep deprivation can cause depression, which in turn further exacerbates sleep problems.

> Sleep deprivation can cause depression, which in turn further exacerbates sleep problems.

The good news is that there is evidence that fixing sleep in new mothers can help with their mood. In one study conducted in the maternity ward at St. Joseph's Healthcare Hamilton, in Canada, by Lori Ross and colleagues, new mothers who were at high risk of developing postpartum depression had the chance to catch up on sleep in the hospital by being given the choice to have a separate room and have their infant spend a few hours in the nursery at night. The 179 mothers enrolled in the study between 1996 and 2001 were at high risk for developing postpartum depression due to either a history of depression or anxiety, or other factors, including socioeconomic influences. After the sleep intervention during their five-day hospital stay, psychiatric admission was lower than typically observed up to two years after giving birth, illustrating the vulnerability of new mothers to sleep deprivation during the perinatal period. Intervening directly with the culprit—baby's sleep—also helps: in an Australian study from 2012, eighty mothers received a forty-five-minute baby sleep consultation, which improved baby's—and thereby mom's—sleep at night—and significantly alleviated feelings of stress, anxiety, and depression.

While most studies evaluating sleep and mood postpartum focus on mothers, more recent studies also investigated paternal sleep and mood patterns. Just like mothers', fathers' sleep is shortened after the baby's birth, albeit sleep fragmentation—usually equivalent to night wakings—occurs at a lower rate in fathers. Importantly, baby's poor sleep is associated with depressive symptoms in fathers too.

In summary, sleep and mood are inseparable. A new baby doesn't sleep well, which disrupts mother's sleep, which worsens her mood, which can lead to baby blues and postpartum depression, which disrupts sleep even more. A two-pronged approach helps break this negative feedback loop: helping the mother and helping the baby—both, together—seems like the most powerful approach to improve well-being and mental health in new mothers.

I can certainly speak to that from my own experience, as well as from coaching families on baby sleep. Being sleep deprived is considered part of the job of a new mother, and often when I pick up the phone to talk to a new mom about sleep, I hear pure desperation in her voice. As a baby sleep coach and mom afflicted by insomnia and mood problems, I believe it's not just important to help parents by helping their babies sleep through the night. As a society we need to recognize the toll sleep deprivation often takes on mothers' mood and normalize the idea of seeking out help from mental health professionals, which need to be readily available. Only in this fashion can we truly attempt to restore a mother's sense of well-being.

The Parental Brain during Sleep Training

I am going into much detail about the physiological and psychological changes we experience after baby's birth because I want to prepare you for discomfort—psychological and even bodily discomfort, when your baby cries because he wants you to come and comfort him at 3 a.m. News alert: It. Does. Not. Feel. Good. Baby's crying presses our alarm button, and the amygdala gets activated and jump-starts parental behaviors, especially for mom: as if on autopilot, your body is summoned to go get your baby and feed him.

It's very, very hard to withstand such internal pressure, especially in a state of sleep deprivation, which affects cognitive function and

HOW BABIES SLEEP SUCCESS STORY:
Mom Brain

One mom I worked with, Helena, told me from the start that she was not going to try any cry-it-out method, because she believed it would cause harm to her four-month-old son, Alexander. I explained to her the research showing that slightly delaying responding to baby's cries—by only ninety seconds!—teaches baby to self-soothe, and even much longer "extinction" sleep training has been shown to not affect children's emotional or cognitive development, even years later. Still, she was too afraid to do it. So finally we talked about her experience when Alexander is crying, and how unbearable that is for her. She told me she feels like Alexander needs her urgently in those moments, and that she cannot refuse him this emotional support. I explained how research shows that babies do not sustain long-term harm from being left to cry, even for much longer than ninety seconds, but how mom's brain is hypersensitized to baby's cries—and that sleep deprivation puts mothers at increased risk for developing depression. Slowly but surely, Helena allowed herself to let go, and to stand Alexander's crying for a few minutes when he woke up at night. Within two nights, Alexander's sleep markedly improved, and he was routinely sleeping six hours at night—to his tired mother's delight.

emotional regulation as described on page 143. Yet it's so powerful to dissociate this internal pressure from real-life consequences of baby's crying. Yes, you feel bad when baby is crying, and your whole brain is firing like crazy trying to get you to tend to her. That's our biological imperative. What I'm asking you to do, right now as well as in that moment, is to consider baby as a separate entity from you. Yes, you feel horrible and *feel* like baby must feel horrible, causing overwhelming empathy. But what if she isn't feeling that horrible, at least not for long? We're not letting her cry for hours, just ninety seconds. Consider how quickly she calms down after you go in. If baby were seriously distraught, she would not settle instantly upon being picked up.

Focus on the fact that baby settles so easily after you go in. Resist the compulsion to go and get baby. Envision a near future where baby won't cry at all at night anymore, and how much less stressful that will be for baby, and you. In my experience as a baby sleep coach, this aspect is the hardest part of sleep training: hearing your baby cry. While I was able to help most parents overcome their intense fear of harming baby by letting her cry for a few minutes, teaching everyone that *It Will Be Fine*, there were a few mothers whose distress became so great as soon as baby started crying that sleep training was too difficult to work. Most mothers I worked with were able to modulate their own emotional response to baby's calls of distress. I explained to them that waiting for a minute and a half is mostly about ourselves as mothers, calming ourselves, setting boundaries for our own behavior, and trying to overcome our mom brain.

> Resist the compulsion to go and get baby. Envision a near future where baby won't cry at all at night anymore, and how much less stressful that will be for baby, and you.

TEACH YOUR BABY TO SLEEP THROUGH THE NIGHT
Key Points

★ Look for signs that your baby is ready to sleep train: he weighs more than eleven pounds, is not too hungry during night feeds, and has slept five to six hours in a stretch at night.

★ Delaying response to your crying baby by just one and a half minutes teaches baby self-soothing.

★ Sleep regression is often a sign to shorten or cut naps.

★ Understand how sleep deprivation and your natural physiological reaction to baby's cries affect you so that you can sleep train effectively.

★ Consider the beneficial effects of sleeping through the night for your mood and well-being.

Solving Common Sleep Problems

Now you know (almost) everything I know about sleep. You've read about circadian rhythms and sleep science, about the importance of entrainment by light, about how schedules help baby sleep and that too much napping makes it hard for baby to feel tired at night.

Using Gentle Sleep Training, we found a way to make the dreaded sleep training less stressful for you, even though, as I explained, it will still be difficult because of the physiological changes in your mom (and dad) brain. But sticking with it will pay off big time, and fast. You know the How Babies Sleep theory; now let's practice. Let's solve your baby's sleep problems together. In this part we will clear up some of the confusion in the baby sleep community—we know better now! You will go through some of the most common baby sleep problems and apply our How Babies Sleep method to solve them.

The questionnaire in "Your How Babies Sleep Solution" (see page 188) will help you develop a specific plan for your baby's sleep schedule.

Chapter 19

Misconceptions about Baby Sleep

Now that you have learned why napping too much and normal light in the evening is bad and how to schedule baby's sleep times, you are in a good position to try to reclaim your nighttime sleep. However, what about all those other sleep coaches and baby sleep books out there? What about the myriad blogs and newsletters you read on the topic, not to mention your friends and own mother, all of whom have an opinion on the subject matter? There is a lot of conflicting advice in the parenting, pediatric, and baby sleep communities. Some of the advice is right, some of it doesn't matter, and some of it is wrong. While we don't understand every aspect of baby's sleep, there are solid ground rules that have been established by scientific research regarding sleep and daily rhythms. After reading this book you will have developed an understanding of the physiological basis for sleep and will hopefully be able to apply this new knowledge to baby's sleep. Our new paradigm, How Babies Sleep, is revolutionary in its approach and simplicity. Let's revisit some of the most common notions about baby sleep and put them in the context of sleep science. For each claim and my discussion of it, I've added the references to the chapter where my reasoning is explained in depth, just in case you want to read more or refresh your memory.

Claim: "All babies are different."

Light affects all humans the same way, allowing entrainment of the circadian clock promoting wakefulness and suppressing melatonin (see chapter 2). Restricting regular light at night is likely to help most babies sleep at night (see chapter 5). While total daily sleep needs are somewhat variable among babies of the same age, all babies continuously sleep less as they get older (see chapter 3). Restricting daytime sleep predictably prolongs nighttime sleep in all babies (see chapter 10).

Claim: "Sleep begets sleep."

"If he sleeps a lot during the day, he will sleep better at night." Wrong! Baby has a total daily sleep need, and if most of that is covered during the day, he will not sleep as much or as well at night. See chapter 10 for details.

Claim: "Imposing a rhythm on baby is unhealthy."

Scientific research shows that our circadian rhythm evolved to help us anticipate changes in our environment. By establishing a feeding and sleep schedule for baby, we are helping her to organize her body and understand and efficiently respond to feelings of fatigue and hunger. Instead of crying inconsolably because she feels unhappy, baby will know she is tired and that it's time to sleep, and she will fall asleep easily. Having set feeding times helps baby's body to be optimally prepared for digestion. Her gastrointestinal tract will anticipate feeding times and start releasing digestive enzymes that quickly and efficiently absorb nutrients. A rhythm gives your baby the much-needed structure she needs to be healthier and happier (see chapter 4).

Claim: "Light doesn't matter."

Most parents do not take enough care to prevent light from coming into the nursery in the early morning hours, and virtually no parents use red light to help baby transition to bedtime or have a strict regular light ban in the nursery. While these are the easiest changes to implement, they have a strong and immediate effect on baby's and toddler's sleep. Using red light at night will help baby fall asleep, and the absence of morning light in his room will keep him asleep until a reasonable hour that works with your schedule (see chapters 2 and 5).

Claim: "Keeping baby awake is unhealthy."

There is no harm in stretching babies' awake time between naps or putting them down later at night at times of transition, so long as you don't make dramatic changes. When we are working on cutting nap times or dropping naps, and we want baby to stay awake a little longer, it's fine to play with him a bit more or carry him around to soothe him before putting him down. A toddler who recently started daycare will be more tired in the evening. You can try moving bedtime earlier; if he consistently falls asleep earlier and still sleeps through the night, the earlier bedtime works. However, if he is just tired on one particular evening, try to stick it out and give him some attention and a long bath, and do other things to keep him happy until his usual bedtime (see chapter 16). Of course, use your judgment and intuition here. You don't want your child to get too irritated to calm down or fall asleep, but stretching awake time by fifteen to thirty minutes for a baby and up to one hour for a toddler or older child should not be a problem (see chapter 10).

Claim: "You should never wake a sleeping baby."

As long as baby's total sleep need is met (and she isn't sick or tired for another reason), you can wake her up at her morning wake time or from a nap to avoid endless napping. This will help create a robust schedule and promote better and longer sleep at night, as she will be more tired (see step 2).

Chapter 20

Common Sleep Problems—and Their Solutions

It is time to put all your newly acquired knowledge to the test and apply the principles of sleep and circadian rhythm to baby's schedule and sleep. Here are the most common issues parents encounter and their solutions.

Baby decides that she wants to get up and play or nurse in the middle of the night

One of the most common problems parents face is that baby gets up too early. When baby is awake at 5 a.m. and wants to start the day, it's hard to stay firm and try to get her to sleep. Parents succumb to their tots' wishes and grudgingly start the day at this ungodly time, hoping that this too shall pass and normal sleep is on the horizon. Unfortunately, they are wrong. By indulging their baby's whim, they are in fact entraining baby's circadian rhythm to a wake time of 5 a.m.

Instead, if your baby wakes too early, try to get her back to sleep. Keep everything dark and only the red light on, speak quietly, rock her, shush her, if necessary pick her up and carry her around. Nurse her a little only if you must, and put her back in her crib. Stay consistent, and after a few days your baby will understand that nighttime is for sleeping, and will wake up by herself at your designated wake time. The most important advice to follow is to keep the room dark and only the red light if needed. Soothe baby, but don't stay in the room too long—you want to indicate that it's time to sleep. If baby doesn't calm down, go back to soothe her again, and leave again. If baby wants to nurse but you know it's only for comfort and she is not really hungry, resist the urge to feed her. For many mothers it is psychologically very difficult not to nurse a crying baby who is visibly upset. What can help in this case is sending in your partner to placate her. Your partner will find another way to calm baby, and she will not be able to insist on nursing.

> The most important advice to follow is to keep the room dark and only the red light if needed.

Keep the wake time constant and open the shades only at the designated wake time. This will likely require a few rough nights, where you go back to the nursery every few minutes to calm a crying baby who wants to party at 5 a.m., but it will pay off very quickly—if you stick to the plan. If she continues to wake up too early, examine her daytime napping. Try shortening her overall daytime sleep duration. Increasing her sleep pressure at night will likely help her sleep better through the night.

Baby has trouble going down at night

You might be tempted to interpret baby's inability to fall asleep as a sign that his bedtime is too early or too late. That is the wrong approach. You set the bedtime according to the sleep times laid out on page 76, and your job is to help him go to bed at that time by entraining his clock through strict repetition and increasing his sleep pressure by adjusting daytime naps. If he cries for hours every night before falling asleep, chances are he is tired but has been napping too much during the day and can't fall asleep because he is not tired enough. Examine his daytime naps on the baby sleep chart on page 30. If they are around or above average sleep amounts for his age, try cutting them to see if that helps with going to bed and sleeping at night (see chapter 10). As your baby grows, you may need to adjust bedtime by an hour or so too.

Baby has trouble going down for her nap

If this keeps happening despite strong entrainment, she might have outgrown this particular nap and be ready to drop it. See chapter 15 on how to drop a nap. If she is consistently extremely tired and fussy after skipping this nap, or even falls asleep in random locations and at random times later on those days, she is probably not ready to skip the nap. Go back to entraining her to a particular nap time and use sleep aids to help her sleep (see chapter 7 for sleep aids). Timing might be another issue. Baby might be able to stay awake longer between naps, so try to move nap time back by half an hour. If the difficult nap is the afternoon nap after lunch, it helps to finish her meal with milk, which has sleep-inducing properties, and to put her down right after. A full tummy will help her go to sleep.

Baby is tired and fussy one day, but it's not bed or nap time yet

This will happen more often with younger babies, before you've firmly established a schedule. It will also happen at times of change in your baby or toddler's life, like after starting daycare, after a move, after the arrival of a new sibling, or while on vacation. Put him down if he is too fussy to be entertained, but try to stick to the schedule as closely as possible. This is especially true for evening bedtime.

How long you can distract baby by playing or carrying her around or other means depends on the baby's age. Very young babies won't be able to stay awake for more than fifteen to thirty minutes when they start being tired. The more closely you are able to repeat nap times every day, the better baby's clock will be entrained, and the easier it will be for baby or toddler to go to sleep at set times. If he consistently remains tired earlier than before, he might be going through a growth spurt, or might be more tired because of a change in his life like starting daycare. Try putting him to bed thirty minutes to one hour earlier. If it doesn't affect nighttime sleep and morning wake time, he might need more sleep.

Baby or toddler skipped a nap and is tired

This is particularly an issue with older babies and toddlers who don't need a specific nap every day anymore and will be tired when they skip their nap. It's tempting to put the cranky kid to bed earlier. Try to stay as close to her usual bedtime as possible, without baby or toddler becoming too fussy. If you put her down too early she might wake up too early, and might be even more tired the next evening. Stick to the schedule to keep a strong rhythm and proper phase alignment.

Baby is tired in the evening, but his bedtime is hours away

If you want baby's longest sleep to be the nighttime sleep when you are sleeping, too, you cannot put baby down too early at night. Many moms will say, "But he's so tired at seven p.m., how do I keep him awake?" This is where your knowledge of the circadian rhythm will come in handy. He's tired at 7 p.m., so put him down for a catnap, but keep the lights bright, don't do your bedtime routine, don't swaddle him, don't use white noise, and don't give him the impression that it's nighttime. No red light, no whispering. If he naps outside his nursery and/or crib during the day, then this nap, too, should happen outside his nursery or crib. Don't be too quiet once he sleeps, so when he wakes up he understands it's still daytime. This behavior will help baby distinguish between naps and nighttime sleep. He won't sleep too long at 7 p.m., and will have another wake phase before it's time for bed. Now at 10 p.m., when you're putting him down for the night, you're going to do the whole bedtime routine, including bath, nursing in his nursery, red light, whispering, and carrying around, and this will signal to baby that it's bedtime. By repeating this every day at the same time, you will entrain baby to a nap time at 7 p.m. and a bedtime of 10 p.m.

SOLVING COMMON SLEEP PROBLEMS
Key Points

★ Most baby sleep advice is not based on science.

★ Scientific evidence provides clear guidelines to help babies sleep.

Weekends, Vacations, and Time Zone Changes

I hope that you're convinced of the great power of creating the right lighting environment for baby, along with setting a proper routine and schedule for baby. But you're probably wondering about how to handle those times when you're away from home and everything is different. What if you're traveling with baby? What about weekends, holidays, and vacations?

Chapter 21

Weekends and Vacations

Many parents report putting babies or older kids to bed later and letting them sleep in on weekends or while on vacation, because they themselves go to bed later and enjoy sleeping longer in the morning when possible. This is problematic for two reasons: it entrains baby's rhythm to a different—later—phase, and it is likely to affect the sleep balance between daytime and nighttime sleep (see chapter 21). Saturdays are often hard for babies and young children because the parents who work during the week are home, weekday caregivers are absent, and nursery school is closed. Mondays are hard because of the transition back to the weekday schedule. On weekends, children are not only in the care of their parents most of the time, they also do different things and go to other places than on weekdays. On vacation these changes are exacerbated, and everything the child knew as normal is upended. That's why children, especially toddlers, often act out

> Keeping schedules the same between weekdays and weekends as well as on vacation helps children adjust.

on weekends and on vacation. It's hard for them that everything is different, and they need time to process these transitions.

Keeping schedules the same between weekdays and weekends as well as on vacation helps children adjust. Knowing what will happen next provides them with a sense of security. The power of How Babies Sleep lies in its robustness. If you put baby down later one day or let him sleep in one day, this will not affect his sleep and happiness too much. However, make the exception an exception.

Of course, I realize that it isn't always possible to follow this program to a T when you're away from home. Sometimes you will arrive in your hotel room, vacation home, grandparents' house, etc. and realize that your hard-earned baby sleep achievements will be put to the test because there is no easy way to block light from the kids' room in the morning. Try your best, be creative, use walk-in closets if you have to as impromptu nurseries. Stuff blankets over curtain rods as DIY blackout shades. Get some actual portable shades or a blackout crib cover (see Baby Travel Sleep Items box). Use other furniture to create a dark corner for the crib. Put baby in the basement if it's safe and you can still hear her if she cries at night. Do what you can to create a dark sleeping environment for baby. Because if you don't, the inevitable will happen, and very fast: baby will wake up earlier—just after sunrise, to be precise. If there is nothing to be done about the light situation, you will at least know what to expect. Instead of repeatedly and frustratingly expecting baby to sleep as long as she does at home, know that she's going to wake earlier on this trip because the morning light reset her clock to an earlier wake-up time. If sunrise isn't too painfully early, it makes sense for the whole family to wake up earlier and consequently go to bed earlier as well.

For bedtime, bring a red light bulb! Your child is entrained to having red light at bedtime, and if he sleeps with the red light, he will protest sleeping in the dark when away from home. The solution? Swap out the bulbs in your hotel room or wherever you're staying. Exchange a light bulb in the room baby sleeps in with the red light bulb you brought. Voilà! Circadian entrainment away from home, including optimal melatonin release at bedtime. Sweet dreams!

Baby Travel Sleep Items
(see page 193 on where to source them)

- -

- Red light bulb

- Portable blackout shades

- Portable crib cover

- White noise machine

- White noise app

Chapter 22

Travel across Time Zones

My kids just turned three and five and I still haven't done any cross-continental travel with them, and haven't visited my home country, Germany, with the kids. Why? Because I'm mortally afraid of how jet lag will upend their carefully calibrated sleep schedules. Don't get me wrong—there are few things I want more than to visit Berlin, my sister, and my parents, or to travel around Europe with my little ones. But knowing how hard jet lag is on myself, I have little desire to spend a week with two jet-lagged toddlers who are fussy from being off their schedules, turning mom into a sleep-deprived zombie.

Let me tell you a little story about jet lag. For that I need to take you on a trip through time and space, to my final year of graduate school. The place: Munich; the year: 2011. After five years of sometimes exhilarating but mostly grueling bench work in the lab, I was exhausted, frustrated, and ready for it to be over so I could move on with my life. The silver lining, the thing that kept me going through hours, days, and weeks of often failing experiments, was my plan to travel after graduating. Travel not to Berlin, or Rome, but to Asia. Far, far away. To escape, to get perspective, to find myself. Not just for a week or two, but for a month, maybe two.

So when I finally passed my doctoral cross-examination in February 2012 and was officially Dr. Axelrod, I did it. I planned a whirlwind of a trip, with all that pent-up wanderlust, exploring not one or two but four countries in six weeks. For the first leg of the trip, I went with my mom to Vietnam and Cambodia, countries I had always dreamed of visiting. The twelve-hour flight from Germany to Hanoi was off to a bad start, made longer because of bad fog and a diverted flight plan. By the time we got to Hanoi—imperial capital of old Vietnam, Paris of the East by way of French colonialism, and modern metropolis of twenty-first-century Asia—I realized I had a problem. I had ambitiously booked a trip with daily excursions, yet I was immediately handicapped by a debilitating condition: jet lag. I really wanted to get up at 5 a.m. and go look at the royal palace from a thousand years ago—and I did—but my body did not feel up to it. I could not sleep at night, because I was still on German time, and I was exhausted. Constantly. For the first week in Vietnam I felt miserable: dizzy and in a terrible mood. When we got to our next stop in Hoi An, I had to stay in the hotel room and sleep until I felt better.

 HOW BABIES SLEEP SUCCESS STORY:
Jet Lag

I had helped Amelia's parents when she was three months old, which had resulted in a blissful ten hours of nighttime sleep for the whole family. When Amelia was four and a half months old, the family flew from New York to Los Angeles, where Amelia's sleep took a turn for the worse. She suddenly started waking up at 2 a.m., and was wide awake at 4 a.m., and she really fought napping. Upon returning after a week, mom Julie was hoping Amelia's sleep would go back to normal, but the baby continued to wake up around eight times at night, was difficult to soothe and crying "hysterically," and was awake—and crying—for a two-and-a-half-hour block in the middle of the night. Julie held off feeding her, and placated her in her crib instead, picking her up when she got very upset. Julie also told me she had gone back to work a few days before, and she was wondering if that might contribute to Amelia's bad sleep. Furthermore, Amelia was teething.

Traveling across time zones is challenging for baby's sleep because being exposed to light and activity at unusual times leads to circadian confusion, also called jet lag. Los Angeles is three hours behind New York, and this abrupt change in bedtime, wake time, and daily activity wreaked havoc on Amelia's sleep. Instead of a strong rhythm and high levels of melatonin in the evening and at night, the prolonged light exposure at night erased the melatonin and confused her clock. At a time when she would normally get up, 5 a.m. New York time, it was only 2 a.m. LA time, when she was expected to sleep.

For short trips, under one week, I recommend keeping baby on the original time zone, especially if the time difference is only three hours. That means Amelia's 7 p.m. New York bedtime becomes 4 p.m. bedtime, and her 5 a.m. wake time turns into a 2 a.m. wake time. Seems crazy? It might be, but this will be the easiest solution to avoid jet lag and bad sleep. You need only one condition to be able to maintain New York rhythm in LA: blackout shades, so that a 4 p.m. bedtime is possible.

If staying on New York time is too impractical, slowly transition baby to LA time, by changing her schedule by one hour a day even before you leave. That means a 5 p.m. bedtime the first day, 6 p.m. bedtime the second day, and so on. This still will be difficult, but not as chaotic and disruptive as trying to shift her by three hours at once, which results in lots of crying. After getting back to New York, the parents can do the same thing in reverse. If Amelia was shifted to LA time, her 7 p.m. bedtime is now 10 p.m. New York time, so shift her back by only one hour a day, so her body has time to adjust. Now that her rhythm has been disrupted, it's back to basics. Entraining her rhythm back to New York time can take up to one week, and it's paramount the light environment and schedules stay exactly the same day after day.

It may seem like jet lag is the cause of Amelia's regression, but it's just part of the story. As is so often the case in life, many things change at once, and it is difficult to differentiate cause from coincidence. I hope this book helps you distinguish the two from each other. Looking at the baby sleep chart on page 30, a four-and-a-half-month-old should sleep no more than three hours during the day, so we need to limit Amelia's daytime sleep, which currently totals four hours per day. Furthermore, to move the 5 a.m. wake time later, she needs to go down later. The baby sleep chart tells us when: for a desired 7 a.m. wake time, put Amelia down ten to ten and a half hours earlier, at 9 p.m.; then she will be able to sleep in longer.

Keeping a tight schedule as well as strict Night Mode and Day Mode will slowly help with jet lag, but it can take up to a week to entrain Amelia's rhythm again. The final step is to go back to Gentle Sleep Training to stop Amelia's night wakings. As Amelia's rhythm gets well entrained to New York time again and she is more tired at night, she will quickly sleep through the night again and regain her confidence in sleeping. After her parents implemented the new schedule at home, Amelia's sleep returned to normal after only one week.

While my trip took a turn for the better after I slept and adjusted to local time, this whole experience—being on an exotic trip but feeling miserable—was quite traumatic. Had I known then what I know now (I started my postdoctoral work in Mike Young's lab studying sleep and circadian rhythms six months later), I could have avoided this forced asynchrony between inner and outer clock, but thankfully I lived to tell you all how to do that.

Based on what we know today about the circadian clock and jet lag, I developed a method to avoid or at least minimize the discomfort associated with crossing time zones. I have personally tested this method in my own family and successfully instructed parents I worked with in its implementation. It is also important to mention that the same method should be applied to situations where you're not going anywhere, but your family or children need to get on a new schedule, for example when they are starting school, or during the transitions from standard to daylight saving time or the other way around.

Given everything I know—and you know, too—it's pretty clear how we can minimize jet lag and sleepless nights. But first, let's revisit what we learned about phase shifts in chapter 2, because that's really all that happens when we travel across time zones:

- Our inner clock is entrained to a twenty-four-hour rhythm.
- Black and white light shifts the clock, but red light doesn't.
- Everything we do or don't do either reinforces or weakens the clock.
- Phase shifts temporarily weaken the rhythm, which disturbs sleep.

Based on these facts, the solution is to not phase shift too abruptly. To understand how to pace this shift, we need to discuss how light resetting works.

After discovering the clock genes named *period* and *timeless*, two of the core clock genes in *Drosophila* flies, my mentor, Mike Young, asked an important question: How do light pulses at different times of the day and night affect the flies' rhythm? To answer this question, fruit flies were exposed to ten-minute light pulses at different times of day and night. After the light pulse, the flies' behavior was monitored for multiple days to determine whether the light had phase shifted their rhythm, and by how much. It turned out that a one-time ten-minute light pulse was sufficient to shift the flies' phase—to induce artificial jet lag, so to speak.

When the flies were exposed to light just after they went to sleep, as if their day was longer than normal, or as if traveling west, their behavioral rhythm became delayed. Conversely, light in the early morning, before dawn, advanced their phase, similar to traveling east. What is interesting about the data is that the magnitude of shifts is not equal between delays and advances. Singular pulses of evening light can cause a phase delay by up to 3.6 hours, but the maximum shift induced by morning light can only reach 2 hours. When pretty much the same experiments were repeated years later with humans, the results were astounding: not only did humans—just like flies—change their rhythmicity in response to light, delaying the phase of their rhythm after evening light exposure and advancing after morning light, but the magnitude of phase shifts was identical between flies and humans. Just like in flies, evening light exposure in humans can cause phase delays up to 3.6 hours, but morning light exposure causes advances of only up to 2 hours, maximum.

> Just like in flies, evening light exposure in humans can cause phase delays up to 3.6 hours, but morning light exposure causes advances of only up to 2 hours, maximum.

Next summer our family wants to travel from New York to Berlin. How do we do that using my method in order to minimize jet lag? We're traveling east, which means we need a phase advance—and that's only happening at a rate of around two hours per day maximally. New York to Berlin is a six-hour time difference, and instead of just flying there and dealing with circadian chaos caused by jet lag, we will do two things:

1. "Travel east" while still in New York
2. "Stay west" while in Berlin

How does this make sense? It's very simple: before traveling to Germany, the whole family will gradually advance our rhythm by a few hours, as much as is convenient with our daily rhythm. One to two hours should be doable.

Starting a week in advance, we will get up an hour earlier than usual, and go to bed an hour earlier—for example 8 p.m. instead of the regular 9 p.m. Then, the last days before the flight, we will get up two hours earlier and go to bed two hours earlier than usual. Now we're already a third of the way between New York and Berlin, somewhere in the Atlantic Ocean, time zone–wise. Flights to Germany are usually red-eye flights overnight, which causes the worst jet lags because of the time shift plus the sleep deprivation. By shifting before the flight we'll have a chance of actually sleeping on the plane, because our rhythm will be more adjusted to an earlier bedtime. If we have our pick of different overnight flights, we should pick one that leaves later, closer to our bedtime. Leaving around 5 p.m. is the worst, because the flight takes around eight hours and will land around 1 a.m. New York time, a time when most of us would have been asleep for just a few hours, but which is 7 a.m. Berlin time. If you even manage to sleep in those uncomfortable planes before 1 a.m., you will have slept for only two hours or so—but then you land and it's morning in Berlin and time to get up. The sleep deprivation plus the morning light make for a highly unpleasant combination.

Upon arriving in Berlin, we'll keep shifting, slowly, by two hours a day. That means for the kids, the bedtime on the first night is not 9 p.m. Berlin time, which is 3 p.m. New York time, but 11 p.m. Berlin time, which is 7 p.m. New York time and 9 p.m. Somewhere-in-the-Atlantic time—our current time zone. Wake-up time on the second day is not 8 a.m. Berlin time, which is 4 a.m. Somewhere-in-the-Atlantic time, but 11 a.m., which is 7 a.m. Somewhere-in-the-Atlantic time, and that night we can fully switch to Berlin time and go to bed at 9 p.m., and get up at 8 a.m. the next day. Voilà, phase shift in three days from New York to Berlin time and no jet lag!

Make sure to keep baby's naps on the same intermediate schedule as the bed and wake times. Your best friends during these transition times, while your rhythm is still misaligned with the local time, are a red light bulb and portable blackout shades (see page 193). You'll need both in the morning, when you want to sleep in to prevent the light of your new time zone from wreaking havoc on your clock.

If traveling for only a few days, I wouldn't bother fully switching to local time. You can use your schedule and manipulate the light conditions with the red light and blackout shades to help stay in your original time zone. Or you may prefer to adjust to an intermediate time zone to avoid

> If traveling for only a few days, I wouldn't bother fully switching to local time.

double jet lag (on the way there and the way back), especially if you're traveling for pleasure and don't have to follow any particular meeting schedule.

If you travel for more than, say, five days, it makes sense to fully switch to the new time zone for days 3–5, and then adjust back to your original time zone before your flight: delay your bedtime by one to two hours, get up later the next day, and again a few days before the flight. Remember, phase delays are easier than phase advances! This means it's easier for us to return to New York from Berlin than to go east to begin with. After arriving in New York, it will only take us another day or two to fully switch to New York time.

Before traveling, write out a phase shift schedule for naps, meals, bedtimes, and wake times for each time zone and each intermediate step. While this seems like a lot of work, and theoretically "going with the flow" appears to be a more natural way to handle jet lag, the planning will pay off when your kids will sleep at night while you're traveling and back at home, allowing you to enjoy your trip and settle back into your routine at home without any travel-induced sleep drama.

> Before traveling, write out a phase shift schedule for naps, meals, bedtimes, and wake times for each time zone and each intermediate step.

Of course, the same is true when traveling west. A week or so before traveling, delay bedtime for yourself and the kids by one hour and get up an hour later, and then closer to the flight by another hour. This is usually more difficult to make work with our schedules (most of us can't roll into work an hour later), but do as much as you can. On overnight flights, use the flight time to your advantage. Delay sleeping on the flight by watching a movie or two; this way you can shift en route and are halfway there in terms of jet lag when you arrive. Make sure not to stay up for more than three hours later than your previous bedtime. When you arrive at your destination, say, Beijing, which for your body is eleven hours behind (or twelve during daylight saving time), try to delay going to bed by no more than three hours for the kids. Everything else will cause circadian chaos. That means, for a normal bedtime of 9 p.m., progressive bedtimes of 1, 4, 7, and then 9 p.m. Bring those blackout shades to make it dark, and put the kids to sleep (see "Baby Travel Sleep Items" box on page 169 for other items to bring). The next morning—which is still middle of the night by Beijing standards— let yourself and the kids sleep no more than one hour past their scheduled wake time, which is their bedtime plus number of hours of nighttime sleep. So, for my children, who normally sleep eleven hours at night, I let them sleep twelve hours, and have progressive wake-up times of 1, 4, 7, and 8 a.m. Not too bad, in my opinion!

The phase shift is complete in only four days, and no jet lag! It sounds crazy to be starting the day in the middle of the night, but really, it's only crazy for the first day, when I want you to get up at 1 a.m.

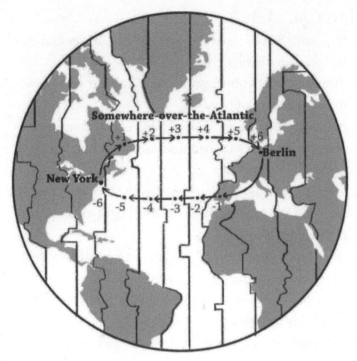

How to Avoid Jet Lag

Before traveling, start transitioning to the time zone you're going to be in. As an example, before traveling from New York to Berlin, start one week before the flight and get up one hour earlier and go to bed one hour earlier. Shift by another hour two days before flying. Now you're not quite on Berlin time, but almost halfway there; you're on Somewhere-in-the-Atlantic time. Upon arrival in Berlin, don't just jump into the local time zone, but keep shifting by no more than two hours a day. That means using blackout shades in the morning to stay on Somewhere-in-the-Atlantic time for another day. After three days you will have fully switched to Berlin time. On the way back, do the same thing in reverse: start going to bed later and getting up later before the flight, and, when back in New York, block out light in the evening to shift by no more than three hours per day (delays are easier on the body than advances, therefore shifts when traveling west is easier and faster than when traveling east).

In my opinion, it's worth having one weird day like that if in exchange you get to have a full "night's" sleep and minimize crying babies.

Here is the jet lag–free recipe for the whole family for travel across time zones:

TRAVELING EAST

1. One week before travel, get up one hour earlier and go to bed one hour earlier.
2. Two days before travel, get up another hour earlier and go to bed another hour earlier.
3. If flying overnight, pick a flight that aligns as much as possible with the kids' bedtime and try to sleep on the plane as soon as you board.
4. When at your destination, shift by no more than two hours per day. Use blackout shades and red light to simulate night in the morning.
5. Four days before the return flight, get up and go to bed an hour later to prepare for home time.
6. Delay baby's naps by no more than one hour, respective to their body's current time zone.
7. Two days before the flight, get up and go to bed another hour later to prepare for your home time zone.
8. After arriving back home, shift back by no more than three hours per day. Use blackout shades and red light to simulate night in the evening.
9. Keep adjusting naps according to the body's current time zone.

TRAVELING WEST

1. One week before travel, sleep one hour later and go to bed one hour later.
2. Two days before travel, get up another hour later and go to bed another hour later.
3. If flying overnight, use the flight time to phase shift by delaying bedtime. For yourself, you can delay up to three hours, for the kids, no more than two hours.
4. When at destination, shift by no more than three hours per day. Use blackout shades and red light to simulate night in the evening.

5. Sleep in later in the mornings by no more than one hour, relative to the body's current time zone.

6. Delay naps by no more than one hour, relative to your body's current time zone.

7. For trips of more than one week: one week before the return flight, get up and go to bed an hour earlier to prepare for your home time zone.

8. For trips of less than one week: shift only as much as three-hour shifts per day get you; if that doesn't get you fully aligned with the local time, don't bother—it's not worth fully switching.

9. Three days before the flight, get up and go to bed an hour earlier to prepare for your home time zone.

10. After returning home, shift no more than two hours per day. Use blackout shades and red light to simulate night in the morning.

11. Keep adjusting naps according to the body's current time zone.

EXAMPLE 1: Flying from New York to Berlin with a two-year-old. Six hours phase advance. Spending seven days in Berlin.

- Regular schedule:
    Wake time ------ *8 a.m.*
    Nap -------------- *1–2 p.m.*
    Bedtime --------- *9 p.m.*

- 1 week before departure:
    Wake time ------ *7 a.m.*
    Nap -------------- *12–1 p.m.*
    Bedtime --------- *8 p.m.*

- 2 days before departure:
    Wake time ------ *6 a.m.*
    Nap -------------- *11 a.m.–12 p.m.*
    Bedtime --------- *7 p.m.*

- Travel day, flight 5 p.m.–1 a.m.:
    Wake time ------ *6 a.m.*
    Nap -------------- *11 a.m.–12 p.m.*
    Bedtime --------- *6 p.m. (should be easy on plane)*

- Day 1 at destination:
    Wake time ------ *7 a.m. (plane lands)*
    Nap -------------- *11 a.m.–2 p.m. (because didn't sleep
                    enough at night)*
    Bedtime --------- *8 p.m.*

- Day 2 at destination:
    Wake time ------ *7 a.m.*
    Nap -------------- *12–1 p.m.*
    Bedtime --------- *9 p.m.*

- Day 3 at destination (home schedule):
    Wake time ------ *8 a.m.*
    Nap -------------- *1–2 p.m.*
    Bedtime --------- *9 p.m.*

- Days 4–5 at destination:
    Wake time ------ *9 a.m.*
    Nap -------------- *2–3 p.m.*
    Bedtime --------- *10 p.m.*

- Day 6 at destination:
    Wake time ------ *10 a.m.*

> *Nap* -------------- *3–4 p.m.*
> *Bedtime* --------- *11 p.m.*

- Day 7, travel day, flight 12–7 p.m.:
    > *Wake time* ------ *10 a.m.*
    > *Nap* -------------- *3–6 p.m. (longer because on plane and to*
    > *allow to push back bedtime due to flight)*
    > *Bedtime* --------- *9 p.m.*

- Day 8, at home:
    > *Wake time* ------ *6 a.m.*
    > *Nap* -------------- *11 a.m.–12 p.m.*
    > *Bedtime* --------- *8 p.m.*

- Day 9, at home:
    > *Wake time* ------ *7 a.m.*
    > *Nap* -------------- *12–1 p.m.*
    > *Bedtime* --------- *9 p.m.*

- Day 10, at home: back to regular schedule

EXAMPLE 2: Flying from New York to Beijing with a two-year-old. Eleven hours phase delay (November to February; twelve hours from March to October because of daylight saving time). Spending fourteen days in Beijing.

- Regular schedule:
    > *Wake time* ------ *8 a.m.*
    > *Nap* -------------- *1–2 p.m.*
    > *Bedtime* --------- *9 p.m.*

- 1 week before departure:
    - *Wake time ------ 9 a.m.*
    - *Nap -------------- 2–3 p.m.*
    - *Bedtime --------- 10 p.m.*

- 2 days before departure:
    - *Wake time ------ 10 a.m.*
    - *Nap -------------- 3–4 p.m.*
    - *Bedtime --------- 11 p.m.*

- Travel day, flight 3:50 p.m.–6:55 p.m.:
    - *Wake time ------ 11 a.m.*
    - *Takeoff ---------- 3:50 p.m. NY time*
    - *Nap -------------- 4–7 p.m. NY time (longer nap because nighttime sleep was cut short)*
    - *Land------------- 6:55 p.m. local time*

- Day 1 at destination:
    - *Wake time ------ 3 a.m.*
    - *Nap -------------- 8–9 a.m.*
    - *Bedtime --------- 4 p.m.*

- Day 2 at destination:
    - *Wake time ------ 6 a.m.*
    - *Nap -------------- 11 a.m.–12 p.m.*
    - *Bedtime --------- 7 p.m.*

- Days 3–9 at destination (home schedule):
    - *Wake time ------ 8 a.m.*
    - *Nap -------------- 1–2 p.m.*
    - *Bedtime --------- 9 p.m.*

- Days 10–11 at destination:
    - *Wake time ------ 7 a.m.*

Nap -------------- *12–1 p.m.*
Bedtime --------- *8 p.m.*

- Days 12–13 at destination:
    Wake time ------ *6 a.m.*
    Nap -------------- *11–12 a.m.*
    Bedtime --------- *7 p.m.*

- Day 14, flight 5 p.m.–7 a.m./6 p.m. local:
    Wake time ------ *5 a.m.*
    Nap -------------- *10–11 a.m.*
    Bedtime --------- *6 p.m.*

- Day 15, flight/at home:
    Wake time ------ *4 a.m./3 p.m. local*
    Nap -------------- *8–9 p.m. local*
    Bedtime --------- *2 a.m. local*

- Day 16, at home:
    Wake time ------ *11 a.m.*
    Nap -------------- *4–5 p.m.*
    Bedtime --------- *12 a.m.*

- Day 17:
    Wake time ------ *9 a.m.*
    Nap -------------- *2–3 p.m.*
    Bedtime --------- *10 p.m.*

- Day 18, regular schedule:
    Wake time ------ *8 a.m.*
    Nap -------------- *1–2 p.m.*
    Bedtime --------- *9 p.m.*

WEEKENDS, VACATIONS, AND TIME ZONE CHANGES
Key Points

★ Keep your kids' schedule the same on weekends as on weekdays.

★ On vacations in the same time zone, keep your regular schedule. Bring portable shades and a red light to help re-create your usual light settings (see "Helpful Baby items" on page 193).

★ When crossing time zones, avoid jet lag by creating a phase shift schedule and slowly shift toward your desired time before, during, and after you travel by no more than three hours per day (two when traveling east).

★ When traveling across time zones, use blackout shades and red light at home and at your destination to gradually shift to a new time zone.

★ Traveling east is harder than traveling west, because phase delays are easier for our bodies than phase advances.

Your How Babies Sleep Solution

You made it! You've stuck with me and made it through this book—congratulations! You are ready to experience your own How Babies Sleep success story, to take the research and advice in these pages and encourage your baby to sleep through the night.

As I hope is clear by now, my goal is not to impose a random set of rules on you, but to foster an informed mind-set, based on the fascinating science of our inner clock and sleep drive, to help you tackle any sleep problem that baby throws your way. This part will help you implement the knowledge from this book and apply it to your baby.

The following questionnaires will guide you through the three steps of my method:

1. Light and Sleep Environment

	Yes	No	Comment
Do you have a red light?			Time to get one! (See page 193 for information on how to source one.)
Do you have blackout shades?			Install permanent or removable blackout shades. (See page 194 for advice on how to source them.)
Does baby sleep in her own crib?			Put her in her own crib—it teaches her self-soothing.
Does baby sleep in her own room?			After two months, put baby in her own room if possible.
Does baby sleep with siblings?			Put the worst sleeper in her own room, so that the rest of the family can get their much-needed rest.

2. Schedule and Naps

	Answer	Comment
When is your preferred wake-up time?		What works best for you and your family?
How old is baby?		If preterm, use corrected age.
What's the recommended total amount of daytime sleep for baby's age?		Check the baby sleep chart on page 30.
Calculate baby's new bedtime.		New bedtime = your desired wake time less baby's recommended hours of nighttime sleep plus buffer time to account for baby's nighttime wakings.

	Answer	Comment
How many naps should baby take?		Check the baby sleep chart on page 30.
How long should baby's naps be in total?		Check the baby sleep chart on page 30.

3. Sleeping through the Night

	Answer	Comment
Does your baby weigh more than eleven pounds?		Babies who weigh more than eleven pounds are usually mature enough to sleep for six or more hours at night.
How old is your baby?		Babies are typically ready for Gentle Sleep Training around three months.
Has your baby ever slept more than five or six hours at night?		Once baby has shown you that she can sleep for five or six hours without feeding, don't backtrack!
When baby wakes up and cries, does she sometimes fall asleep while nursing?		Babies who don't seem that hungry during night feeds are nursing for comfort, not out of hunger. Time to sleep train!

	Answer	Comment
Have you answered yes to all of the questions above?		If no, don't despair. Keep up the light entrainment, work on the schedule and naps, and wait until baby shows signs of readiness before you start Gentle Sleep Training. If yes, congratulations! Baby is ready for sleep training!
How long should I wait before feeding baby during the night?		Calculate how long to wait before feeding baby by taking his longest sleep stretch and subtracting 1 hour.
Baby is crying at night. If it's time to nurse, what do I do?		Nurse baby and put her back in the crib drowsy, but not asleep, and leave the room.
Baby is crying at night. If it's *not* time to nurse, what do I do?		Follow my Gentle Sleep Training method: 1) Wait one and a half minutes before going in to check on baby. 2) Placate baby from the crib. 3) Leave after two to three minutes, even if baby is still crying. 4) Repeat until baby is asleep or it is time to feed.

How Babies Sleep Charts

This chart summarizes the three steps to baby sleep outlined in this book. You can cut it out and put it on your fridge or take a picture of it to keep it handy on your phone.

Three steps to better sleep

1 Light and sleep environment

Babies are senstive to light—at night it reduces the sleep hormone melatonin, in the morning it resets their clock

▷ Red light

▷ Blackout shades

2 Naps and schedule

Babies have a total 24 hour sleep need, which continuously decreases until adulthood

Napping reduces nighttime sleep

▷ Adjust naps according to this chart

▷ Set bedtime according to your desired wake up time

▷ Resisting naps indicates baby needs less sleep. Shorten or cut naps

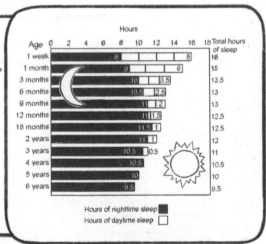

3 Sleeping through the night

Signs of readiness for Gentle Sleep Training:

- Weighs over 11 lbs
- Has ever slept 5+ hours
- Doesn't seem hungry when nursed at night

▷ Use flowchart to guide nighttime sleep training

Use this decision tree to help you during Gentle Sleep Training:

Sleeping through the night

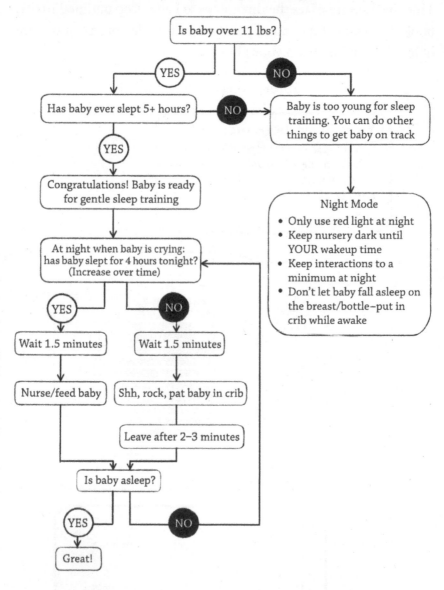

Helpful Baby Items

- For extra support on your sleep training journey, download my **Kulala baby sleep app**, based on the program described in this book. The Kulala app contains most of the info from this book at your fingertips, and is especially helpful in creating and maintaining a schedule for your baby, which is automatically updated as baby gets older. Available at the Google Play store and Apple App Store. Also see the last page.

- **Red light:** This is essential to keep baby in Night Mode. You can find red light bulbs for sale (amazon.com) and can use those bulbs with any lamp that you own. Or order my special Kulala lamp from Kulalaland.com, which is especially engineered to be completely free of wake-promoting blue light, along with other features like silent touch control to not wake baby up and adjustable dimming: Turning on when baby starts crying, touch dimming, and featuring soothing white noise. If you buy red bulbs from somewhere else, get LEDs that emit the equivalent of 60 watts. Not only are they much longer-lived and more energy efficient compared to old-fashioned incandescent bulbs, but their red hue is also "cleaner" and better suited to help babies sleep. With 60 watts you can see well enough to even read a book, and if your toddler wants to sleep with that light, put the lamp in a corner so it's not too bright.

- **Blue light filter apps** for smartphones and computers. iPhones now have a Night Shift mode, and Android phones a Night-Light mode. Program both to automatically turn on two hours before it's baby's bedtime, and turn off at wake time. I recommend installing an additional blue light filter app (there are various ones available in the app stores), as the native ones don't make the screen quite red enough. The screen should look distinctively reddish, not just yellow. Also use Night Shift on Macs and iPads and install a program called f.lux for Windows computers. Program those filters to turn on and off automatically like described about your phone.

- **Blackout shades** are necessary to keep baby in Night Mode until it's *your* desired wake-up time. You have endless options here! You can buy blackout curtains to hang on your window treatments. You can also opt for an easy-to-install adhesive shade like the Bobotogo Black Pleated Blackout shades (amazon.com) or a portable option like the AmazonBasics Portable Baby Travel Window Blackout Blind Shades with Suction Cups (amazon.com).

- **Portable crib covers** are useful during traveling to control light exposure in a hotel room or at Grandma's house. They cover the crib and block out light, while allowing airflow to keep baby safe. One option is the SnoozeShade Pack N Play Crib Canopy and Tent (amazon.com).

- **White noise app:** multiple versions are available in Apple and Google app stores.

- **Baby tracker app:** Many are available for free in the Apple and Google app stores. A tracking app will help you note how often you feed baby, how often baby has diaper changes, and what baby's sleep times looks like. Therefore it can help with establishing schedules.

- **White noise machine:** These help baby sleep, especially if there is a sibling or baby sleeps with parents in the same room. You have lots of purchasing options, like Amazon. Our Kulala baby sleep lamp has it built in (see the last page).

- **Rocking bassinet:** Rocking bassinets are great for soothing baby; the rocking motion calms him down. There are lots of different makes to choose from.

- **Baby swing:** Swings are useful tools for daytime naps. For babies younger than two months, make sure baby lies completely flat and with her chin off her chest to ensure proper breathing. One good brand is the My Little Snugabunny from Fisher-Price (amazon.com).

- **SwaddleMe swaddle blankets:** These are the ultimate sleep aid and are great for helping you swaddle your baby nice and snug overnight when you want him to sleep the longest. They sell for about fifteen dollars for a two-pack on Amazon and are available at other baby product retailers.

- **Sleep sack:** Blankets are not safe for babies, so sleep sacks can add warmth for babies who outgrow swaddling. Various versions are available.

References and Additional Reading

Here are some of the scientific studies I used to formulate my method. If you find a specific topic particularly fascinating, you can find more information below.

Human Circadian Rhythms

Czeisler, C. A., and J. J. Gooley. "Sleep and Circadian Rhythms in Humans." *Cold Spring Harbor Symposia on Quantitative Biology* 72, no. 1 (2007): 579–97. https://doi.org.10.1101/sqb.2007.72.064.
Comprehensive review of human circadian rhythms.

Globig, M. "A World without Day or Night." *MaxPlanckResearch* (2007): 60–61.
Recap of more than thirty years of studying human circadian rhythms in Germany.

Patke, A. et al., "Mutation of the Human Circadian Clock Gene CRY1 in Familial Delayed Sleep Phase Disorder." *Cell* 169, no. 2 (2017): 203–15.e13. https://doi.org.10.1016/j.cell.2017.03.027.
Study from our lab describing the human "night owl gene."

Fly Clock Mutants

Konopka, R. J., and S. Benzer. "Clock Mutants of Drosophila Melanogaster." *Proceedings of the National Academy of Sciences* 68, no. 9 (1971): 2112–16. https://doi.org/10.1073/pnas.68.9.2112.
The first study to describe the existence of genetic mutations that alter the circadian rhythm.

Thaddeus A. Bargiello, F. Rob Jackson, and Michael W. Young. "Restoration of Circadian Behavioural Rhythms by Gene Transfer in *Drosophila.*" *Nature* 312, 752–54 (1984). https://doi.org.10.1038/312752a0.

William A. Zehring, David A.Wheeler, Pranhitha Reddy, Ronald J. Konopka, Charalambos P. Kyriacou, Michael Rosbash, Jeffrey C. Hall. "P-element Transformation with Period Locus DNA Restores Rhythmicity to Mutant, Arrhythmic Drosophila Melanogaster," *Cell* 39, 2 (1984) 369–76. https://doi .org.10.1016/0092-8674(84)90015-1.

These two studies identified the first genes required for rhythmic behavior in the fruit fly, thereby starting the field of molecular chronobiology. The authors, Mike Young, Michael Rosbash, and Jeff Hall, were awarded the Nobel Prize in Medicine or Physiology for these and subsequent findings on the genes comprising the molecular clock.

Light as a Zeitgeber

Lockley, S. W., G. C. Brainard, and C. A. Czeisler. "High Sensitivity of the Human Circadian Melatonin Rhythm to Resetting by Short Wavelength Light." *The Journal of Clinical Endocrinology & Metabolism* 88, no. 9 (2003): 4502. https://doi.org.10.1210/jc.2003-030570.

First study showing that human melatonin rhythms are highly sensitive to blue light.

Green, A. et al., "Evening Light Exposure to Computer Screens Disrupts Human Sleep, Biological Rhythms, and Attention Abilities." *Chronobiology International* 34, no. 7 (2017): 855–65. https://doi.org.10.1080/07420528 .2017.1324878.

Evening exposure to blue but not orange light disrupts sleep and the circadian clock in humans.

Hale, L., and S. Guan. "Screen Time and Sleep among School-Aged Children and Adolescents: A Systematic Literature Review." *Sleep Medicine Reviews* 21 (2015): 50–58. https://doi.org.10.1016/j.smrv.2014.07.007.

Meta-analysis of sixty-seven scientific studies showing that evening exposure to screens is correlated with poor sleep in children.

Akacem, L. D., K. P. Wright Jr., and M. K. LeBourgeois. "Sensitivity of the Circadian System to Evening Bright Light in Preschool-Age Children." *Physiological Reports* 6, no. 5 (2018). https://doi.org.10.14814/phy2.13617.
Exposure to bright light in the evening erases melatonin for hours in toddlers.

Zeitzer, J. M. et al., "Sensitivity of the Human Circadian Pacemaker to Nocturnal Light: Melatonin Phase Resetting and Suppression." *The Journal of Physiology* 526, no. 3 (2000): 695–702. https://doi.org.10.1111/j.1469-7793.2000.00695.x.
Light as dim as candlelight is sufficient to suppress melatonin and reset the clock.

Wyszecki, G., and W. S. Stiles. *Color Science: Concepts and Methods, Quantitative Data and Formulae,* 2nd ed. New York: Wiley & Sons, 2000.
The bible of research into the colors of light and how we perceive them.

Stothard, E. R. et al., "Circadian Entrainment to the Natural Light-Dark Cycle across Seasons and the Weekend." *Current Biology: CB* 27, no. 4 (2017): 508–13. https://doi.org.10.1016/j.cub.2016.12.041.
Release of the sleep hormone melatonin and sleep are delayed by evening light exposure, but can be restored by a weekend camping trip.

Food as a Zeitgeber

Stokkan, K. A. et al., "Entrainment of the Circadian Clock in the Liver by Feeding." *Science* 291, no. 5503 (2001): 490–93. https://doi.org.10.1126/science.291.5503.490.
This important paper shows that food can act as a zeitgeber, entraining rats—and their livers—to a wake time in the middle of the night.

Wehrens, S. M. T. et al., "Meal Timing Regulates the Human Circadian System." *Current Biology: CB* 27, no. 12 (2017): 1768–75.e3. https://doi.org.10.1016/j.cub.2017.04.059.
Eating five hours later than usual causes a metabolic shift.

Damiola, F. et al., "Restricted Feeding Uncouples Circadian Oscillators in Peripheral Tissues from the Central Pacemaker in the Suprachiasmatic

Nucleus." *Genes & Development* 14, no. 23 (2000): 2950–61. https://doi
.org.10.1101/gad.183500.

If the zeitgebers light and food are in conflict, the brain stays on light-time, but the liver switches to food time, causing different time zones to coexist in your body.

White, W., and W. Timberlake. "Two Meals Promote Entrainment of Rat Food-Anticipatory and Rest-Activity Rhythms." *Physiology & Behavior* 57, no. 6 (1995): 1067–74. https://doi.org.10.1016/0031-9384(95)00023-c.

Without light, food can act as a bona fide zeitgeber and entrain behavioral rhythms.

Evanoo, G. "Infant Crying: A Clinical Conundrum." *Journal of Pediatric Health Care* 21, no. 5 (2007): 333–38. https://doi.org.10.1016/j.pedhc.2007.06.014.

Daily schedules can help reduce baby crying.

Sleep in Babies

Galland, B. C. et al. "Normal Sleep Patterns in Infants and Children: A Systematic Review of Observational Studies." *Sleep Medicine Reviews* 16, no. 3 (2012): 213–22. https://doi.org.10.1016/j.smrv.2011.06.001.

Meta-analysis of thirty-four studies reviewing sleep patterns in almost seventy thousand children from eighteen different countries, aged zero to twelve years.

Jenni, O. G., and M. K. LeBourgeois. "Understanding Sleep–Wake Behavior and Sleep Disorders in Children: The Value of a Model." *Current Opinion in Psychiatry* 19, no. 3 (2006): 282–87. https://doi.org.10.1097/01.yco
.0000218599.32969.03.

Review sleep in babies explaining that sleep pressure rises faster in babies than in adults.

Nakagawa, M. et al. "Daytime Nap Controls Toddlers' Nighttime Sleep." *Scientific Reports* 6 (2016). https://doi.org.10.1038/srep27246.

Longer naps during the day directly reduce nighttime sleep duration in young children.

Sleep Disturbances

Kang, J.-H., and S.-C. Chen. "Effects of an Irregular Bedtime Schedule on Sleep Quality, Daytime Sleepiness, and Fatigue among University Students in Taiwan." *BMC Public Health* 9, no. 1 (2009): 201–6. https://doi.org .10.1186/1471-2458-9-248.

Irregular bedtimes negatively affected sleep in Taiwanese college students.

Foster, R. G. et al., "Sleep and Circadian Rhythm Disruption in Social Jetlag and Mental Illness," *Progress in Molecular Biology and Translational Science* 119 (2013) 325–46. https://doi.org.10.1016/B978-0-12-396971-2.00011-7.

Review on the different types of sleep disorders and circadian rhythm disorders, including self-imposed social jet lag.

Baby's Clock

Rivkees, S. A. "Developing Circadian Rhythmicity in Infants." *Pediatrics* 112, no. 2 (2003): 373–81. https://doi.org.10.1542/peds.112.2.373.

Preterm NICU babies that were exposed to light/dark cycles of illumination showed quick entrainment of their sleep/wake cycles, proving that babies can develop circadian rhythmicity if properly entrained.

Kinoshita, M. et al., "Paradoxical Diurnal Cortisol Changes in Neonates Suggesting Preservation of Foetal Adrenal Rhythms." *Scientific Reports* (2016): 1–7. https://doi.org.10.1038/srep35553.

Newborns exhibit reversed twenty-four-hour cycles of cortisol, which mature by two months of age.

Gentle Sleep Training

Ferber, R. *Solve Your Child's Sleep Problems.* New York: Simon & Schuster, 1985, 2006.

Dr. Ferber popularized the idea that babies need to learn self-soothing to sleep through the night. Parents often interfere with that process by forming unnecessary sleep associations in babies, such as being carried around.

Adair, R. et al., "Reducing Night Waking in Infancy: A Primary Care Intervention." *Pediatrics* 89, no. 4, part 1 (1992): 585–88.
Sleep in babies improved after parents were told about how to teach baby to self-soothe.

Conty, L., N. George, and J. K. Hietanen. "Watching Eyes Effects: When Others Meet the Self." *Consciousness and Cognition* 45 (2016): 184–97. https://doi .org.10.1016/j.concog.2016.08.016.
Looking people in the eye increases arousal—therefore don't look directly in baby's eyes when you want her to sleep.

Gerard, C. M., K. A. Harris, and B. T. Thach. "Spontaneous Arousals in Supine Infants while Swaddled and Unswaddled during Rapid Eye Movement and Quiet Sleep." *Pediatrics* 110, no. 6 (2002): e70. https://doi.org.10.1542/ peds.110.6.e70.
Swaddling is highly effective in calming babies.

Spencer, J. A. et al., "White Noise and Sleep Induction." *Archives of Disease in Childhood* 65, no. 1 (1990): 135–37. https://doi.org.10.1136/adc.65.1.135.
White noise helps babies sleep.

Fleming, P., P. Blair, and A. Pease. "Why or How Does the Prone Sleep Position Increase the Risk of Unexpected and Unexplained Infant Death?" *Archives of Disease in Childhood: Fetal and Neonatal Edition* (2017): 1–2. https://doi. org.10.1136/archdischild-2017-313331.
Why stomach sleeping is considered unsafe.

Chen, H.-Y. et al., "Physiological Effects of Deep Touch Pressure on Anxiety Alleviation: The Weighted Blanket Approach." *Journal of Medical and Biological Engineering* 33, no. 5 (2013): 463–70.
How deep-pressure stimulation, including weighted blankets, calms the nervous system, which is probably why stomach sleeping helps some babies sleep.

St. James-Roberts, I. et al., "Video Evidence That Parenting Methods Predict Which Infants Develop Long Night-Time Sleep Periods by Three Months of Age." *Primary Health Care Research & Development* 18, no. 3 (2017): 212–26. https://doi.org.10.1097/DBP.0000000000000166.
Powerful study using video analysis of parents who either cosleep with their

babies or have baby in a separate crib. Parents who delayed responding to baby's crying—simply because baby was not cosleeping with them—by 1–1.5 minutes were more likely to have babies who slept five or more hours at night at three months of age.

Mindell, J. A. et al., "Developmental Aspects of Sleep Hygiene: Findings from the 2004 National Sleep Foundation Sleep in America Poll." *Sleep Medicine* 10, no. 7 (2009): 771–79. https://doi.org.10.1016/j.sleep.2008.07.016.
Bedtime routines help babies sleep.

Volkovich, E. et al., "Sleep Patterns of Co-sleeping and Solitary Sleeping Infants and Mothers: A Longitudinal Study." *Sleep Medicine* 16, no. 11 (2015): 1305–12. https://doi.org.10.1016/j.sleep.2015.08.016.
Cosleeping mothers report more infant night wakings and poorer sleep than mothers of babies who sleep in their own cribs.

Porter, R. H., and J. Winberg. "Unique Salience of Maternal Breast Odors for Newborn Infants." *Neuroscience and Biobehavioral Reviews* 23 (1999): 439–49. https://doi.org.10.1016/s0149-7634(98)00044-x.
Infants are able to recognize and are attracted to the scent of their mother's breast milk.

Jet Lag

Myers, M. P. et al., "Light-Induced Degradation of TIMELESS and Entrainment of the Drosophila Circadian Clock." *Science* 271, no. 5256 (1996): 1736–40. https://doi.org.10.1126/science.271.5256.1736.
Study from our lab showing that changing the timing of light pulses throughout day and night can shift flies' circadian rhythm. Evening light causes phase delays, while morning light causes phase advances.

Khalsa, S. B. S. et al., "A Phase Response Curve to Single Bright Light Pulses in Human Subjects." *The Journal of Physiology* 549, part 3 (2003): 945–52. https://doi.org.10.1113/jphysiol.2003.040477.
Repeat of fruit fly experiments in humans reveals the same responses to light exposure: evening light causes phase delays, morning light causes phase advances.

How Motherhood Changes the Brain

Marlin, B. J. et al. "Oxytocin Enables Maternal Behavior by Balancing Cortical Inhibition." *Nature* 520, no. 7548 (2015): 499–504. https://doi.org.10.1038/nature14402.
Study in mice showing that oxytocin enables maternal behavior—by heightening sensitivity to their pups' crying.

Brunton, P. J., and J. A. Russell. "The Expectant Brain: Adapting for Motherhood." *Nature Reviews Neuroscience* 9, no. 1 (2008): 11–25. https://doi.org.10.1038/nrn2280.
Review describing the neurological, hormonal, and psychiatric changes throughout pregnancy and childbirth.

Lafrance, A. "What Happens to a Woman's Brain when She Becomes a Mother." *The Atlantic* (January 2015). https://www.theatlantic.com/health/archive/2015/01/what-happens-to-a-womans-brain-when-she-becomes-a-mother/384179/.
Great article describing the science behind the joy, love, and anxiety that we experience when we become parents.

Functions of Sleep

Rechtschaffen, A., and B. M. Bergmann. "Sleep Deprivation in the Rat: An Update of the 1989 Paper." *Sleep* 25, no. 1 (2002): 18–24. https://doi.org.10.1093/sleep/25.1.18.
This article summarizes the results of the authors' previous research on total sleep deprivation in the rat, and addresses the remaining uncertainty regarding the function of sleep.

Alhola, P., and P. Polp-Kantola. "Sleep Deprivation: Impact on Cognitive Performance." *Neuropsychiatric Disease and Treatment* 3, no. 5 (2007): 553–67. https://www.ncbi.nlm.nih.gov/pubmed/19300585.
Review on effects of total and partial as well as acute and chronic sleep deprivation on human cognition.

Sleep and Mood

Ross, L. E., B. J. Murray, and M. Steiner. "Sleep and Perinatal Mood Disorders: A Critical Review." *Journal of Psychiatry & Neuroscience* 30, no. 4 (2005): 247–56. https://www.ncbi.nlm.nih.gov/pubmed/16049568.
Comprehensive review of the relationship between sleep and mood in new mothers. Poor sleep in new mothers is associated with low mood, baby blues, and postpartum depression (PPD). Helping new mothers sleep decreases PPD in high-risk mothers.

Montgomery-Downs, H. E., and R. Stremler. "Postpartum Sleep in New Mothers and Fathers." *The Open Sleep Journal* 6, no.1 (2013): 87–97.
In new fathers, too, sleep is disrupted and is associated with increased risk for depression.

Symon, B., M. Bammann, G. Crichton, C. Lowings, and J. Tucsok. "Reducing Postnatal Depression, Anxiety and Stress Using an Infant Sleep Intervention." *BMJ Open* 2, no. 5 (2012). https://doi.org.10.1136/bmjopen-2012-001662.
Helping babies sleep improves depression symptoms in new mothers.

Acknowledgments

Mostly I just want to thank everyone I ever talked to about this project for encouraging me and believing in me. First and foremost, I would like to thank my husband, who always put up with my "scientific parenting," and encouraged me in doing so, probably because of the success rate. He read the first draft and said, "This is really good," sealing the deal for me.

Andreas Keller, my agent/friend/science buddy, has been incredibly helpful and supportive throughout all stages of writing and publishing this book, and I felt like he was all the support I needed when it came to buckling down and finishing it. Sarah Pelz took a chance on me and believed from the start that I could contribute something significant to the crowded baby sleep book community. Her guiding me was wonderful and opened up new avenues I would have not chosen myself. She made me into a baby sleep coach. As my editor at Simon & Schuster, Sarah was also instrumental in bringing this book to its final form, improving aspects of it I didn't even realize could be improved. Special thanks to Melanie Iglesias Pérez and the whole team at Simon & Schuster for bringing this book to life.

Finally I want to thank the mothers and fathers I worked with, who indirectly helped create this book. Working with them has been empowering and confidence building—they made me realize how powerful my method is, and how many people could be helped by using it. By helping them I helped myself, because we shared an experience that could not be more polarizing: the magic of motherhood and endless love for your baby, and the grueling sleep deprivation and self-abandonment that make you feel terrible, but that you cannot really share with anyone. Their sharing it with me was very special, and in some ways healed the wounds I carried from those dark postpartum weeks and months.

Index

A

adaptation, 19

adrenal gland, 138

American Academy of Pediatrics
    (AAP), 54, 62, 63, 98

amygdala, 141, 148

anxiety, 141, 147

apps, 93, 99

    baby tracker, 194–95

    Kulala, 94, 99, 112, 115, 125

Aschoff, Jürgen, 7

B

baby blues, 146–48

baby items, helpful, 193–95

bassinets, rocking, 195

bed-sharing, 63–67

bedtime, 33, 38, 76–78

    inability to fall asleep at,
        160–61

    last nap before, 127

    routine for, 89–91, 90, 100

    tiredness long before, 162–63

Benzer, Seymour, 6–8

birth weight, 73–74, 80

blackout shades, 21, 44, 47–48, 53,
    90, 168, 179, 194

blankets:

    muslin, 62

    SwaddleMe, 195

blue light, 14–17, 15, 16, 19, 44–45,
    47–51, 51, 194

    filter apps for, 194

bonding, xxiii, 138, 140

brain, xvii, xxii

    amygdala in, 141, 148

    eye contact and, 59–60

    hypothalamus in, 138

    parental, 136–51

    sleep deprivation and, 143–45

    suprachiasmatic nucleus in, xviii,
        9, 10, 12, 14–15, 19, 20, 22, 35

    see also hormones

breastfeeding, see nursing

Brown University, 100

bunker experiment, 7

C

California Institute of Technology, 6

camping experiment, 49

candlelight, 19, *20*

caregivers, 133–35

cave experiment, 7

childbirth hormones, 138–39

circadian clock, circadian rhythm,
    xvi, xviii, 3–9, *5,* 11, *13,* 24–25,
    55, 100, 101, 156
  amplitude in, 12, *13,* 36–38
  animal kingdom examples of, 4
  of babies, 38–40, 46
  broken and immature, 32–40
  cave and bunker experiments
      on, 7
  disruption of, 32–35
  entrainment in, xix, 10–11, 12,
      19, 22, 34–36, 39, 57, 59, 87,
      129, 156
  genes in, xiii, xviii, 3, 6, 8–9, 10, 35
  how it works, 6–9
  intrinsically photosensitive
      retinal ganglion cells in, 10,
      12, 14, 19, 20
  light and, 10–23; *see also* light
  phase and phase shifts in, 11–12,
      13, *13,* 14, 19, 34–36
  in plants, 4
  periods in, 11, *13*
  power of, 5–6
  sleep pressure alignment with,
      37
  suprachiasmatic nucleus in, xviii,
      9, 10, 12, 14–15, 19, 20, 22, 35
  travel and, *see* travel across time
      zones
  value of, 35–38

Color Science (Wyszecki and Stiles),
    19

computer, tablet, and smartphone
    screens, 16, 49, 50–51, *51,*
    194

cortisol, *16,* 24–25, 38–39, *51,* 138

cosleeping, 63–67

crankiness, *see* fussiness and
    crankiness

crib, 63–67
  covers for, 194
  transition to bed from, 66

crying, 63, 102, 112, 136, 141,
    149–50, 156, 160
  "cry it out" method of sleep
      training, 56, 149
  Gentle Sleep Training and,
      112–13, *116,* 118, 120, 136
  pacifiers and, 61–62
  schedules and, 75, 76, 101
  siblings and, 68–69
  soothing and, *see* soothing

cryptochrome, 35

Czeisler, Charles, 12

D

darkness:
  blackout shades for, 21, 44, 47–48,
      53, 90, 168, *179,* 194
  constant, 22–23

daycare or nursery school, 133–34,
    157, 161
  naps in, 134–35

daylight, *15, 16,* 18, *20,* 21, 47, 49, *51,*
    52, 157

Day Mode, 46, 52, *53*, 55, 93, 101

depression, 146–49

digestion, 22, 23, 32, 33, 34, 38, 156–57

dopamine, 140

Drosophila melanogaster (fruit flies), xviii, 6–8, 25, 35–37, 43–44, 48, 174–75

E

entrainment, xix, 10–11, 12, 19, 22, 34–36, 39, 57, 59, 87, 129, 156

environment, *see* light and sleep environment

estrogen, 139

evening:
    cluster feeding in, 85–86
    routine in, 89
    tiredness in, 162–63
    see also night

eyes:
    eye contact, 59–60
    intrinsically photosensitive retinal ganglion cells in, 10, 12, 14, 19, 20
    lenses in, 17

F

falling reflex, 58

fathers, 140, 141, 147
    bonding and, 138

Ferber, Richard, 56–57

food, feeding, 38, 46, 73–74
    birth weight and, 73–74, 80

cluster feeding in the evening, 85–86

digestion and, 22, 23, 32, 33, 34, 38, 156–57

eating for comfort rather than hunger, 108

Gentle Sleep Training and, 114–15, 118, 122

naps and, 83

newborns and, 80, 83, 86

nighttime, 19–21, 61, 63, 73, 77, 93, 107

schedules for, 23, 73–76, 78–83, 101, 156

trends in, 101

as zeitgeber (time cue), 11, 22–23, 34

see also nursing

fruit flies, xviii, 6–8, 25, 35–37, 43–44, 48, 174–75

fussiness and crankiness, 23, 75, 87, 102, 161–62
    human pacifier trap and, 86–88
    naps and, 98, 127–28
    witching hour and, 85–86

G

Galland, Barbara, 29, 107

genes, xiii, xviii, 3, 6, 8–9, 10, 35

Gentle Sleep Training, xxi, 44, 57, 65, 85, 88, 93, 108, 110–17, 118–22, 136
    crying and, 112–13, *116*, 118, 120, 136
    decision tree for, *192*

Gentle Sleep Training (*cont.*)
efficacy of, 118
example schedule for three-
month-old, 115
feeding and, 114–15, 118, 122
four steps in, 110–12
and jagged curve to nighttime
sleep, 118, *119*
length of time needed for, 118,
120–21
partner's help in, 120
signs of readiness for, 107–9, *117*
success stories on, 108–9, 113–14,
121, 144
tweaking schedule in, 121–22

H
Hall, Jeff, xiii
Harvard Medical School, 12
helpful baby items, 193–95
hormones, 24, 136–37
in childbirth, 138–39
cortisol, *16*, 24–25, 38–39, *51*,
138
estrogen, 139
melatonin, 15, 16, *16*, 17, 20,
24–25, 34, 36, 39, 45, 49, 50,
51, 52, 156
oxytocin, xx, 138–40
postpartum hormones, 139–42
in pregnancy, xxii, 137–38
progesterone, 138, 139
prolactin, 139
serotonin, *16*, 25, *51*
testosterone, 138

How Babies Sleep method:
adjustments and modification of
guidelines in, xxiv–xxv, 132
chart on three steps to better
sleep, 191
consistency and repetition in,
37, 39
entrainment in, 59, 129
Gentle Sleep Training, *see* Gentle
Sleep Training
how to use this book, xx–xxii
partner and, 135
questionnaires on, 187–90
your How Babies Sleep solution,
187–95
How Babies Sleep success stories,
xix
blackout shades, 48
cosleeping to own room, 65
Gentle Sleep Training, 108–9,
113–14, 121, 144
human pacifier trap, 87–88
jet lag, 171–73
light, 21
mom brain, 149
naps, 27
red light, 44
schedule for a five-month-old,
84–85
schedule for a newborn, 81
shortening naps, 99
sickness, 131
sleep deprivation, 144
sleeping in the stroller, 60
sleep regression, 125–26

human pacifier trap, 83, 86–88

hypothalamic-pituitary-adrenal
    (HPA) axis, 138

I

incandescent light bulbs, 16, 44, 193

Indiana University, 22

intrinsically photosensitive retinal
    ganglion cells (ipRGCs), 10,
    12, 14, 19, 20

intuition, xxii–xxiv, 101, 157

J

jet lag, 12, *13*, 19, 34–36, 126
    avoiding, 179–81, *179*
    success story on, 171–73
    see also travel across time zones

jet lag, social, 33

K

Kleitman, Nathaniel, 7

Konopka, Ron, 6–8

Kulala baby sleep app, 94, 99, 112,
    115, 125, 193

Kulala lamp, 193

L

LeBourgeois, Monique, 17

LEDs, 16, 193

Lee, Kathryn, 146

light, xiii, xix, xx, 156, 157
    absence of, 22–23
    adaptation to, 19
    artificial, 16, 49
    candlelight, 19, *20*

circadian clock and, 10–23; *see
    also* circadian clock, circadian
    rhythm

daylight, sunlight, *15, 16,* 18, *20,*
    21, 47, 49, *51,* 52, 157

entrainment and, xix, 10–11, 12,
    19

intensity of, 11, 12–14, 18–19, *20*

power of, underestimation of,
    18–21, *20*

success story on, 21

time of day exposure to, 11,
    12–14

wavelength of, *see* light color

as zeitgeber, 10, 11, 34

light and sleep environment, xvii–
    xviii, 41–69
    chart on, *191*
    common techniques to calm baby
        and encourage rest, 57–58
    cosleeping in, 63–67
    crib in, 63–67
    Day Mode and, 46, 52, *53,* 55,
        93, 101
    designated space for night sleep,
        60
    eye contact and, 59–60
    helping baby fall asleep, 54–69
    Night Mode and, 46–52, *53,* 55,
        68–69, 76, 77, 89, *90,* 91, 93,
        101, 129
    pacifiers and, 61–62
    questionnaire on, 188
    red light in, 43–45; *see also* red
        light

light and sleep environment (*cont.*)
  safety and, 54–55
  self-soothing and, 56–57
  siblings and, 67–69
  swaddling in, 58–59
  where the baby sleeps, 63–67
  white noise in, 61, 68, 194, 195
light bulbs, incandescent, 16, 44, 193
light color (wavelength), 11, 14–17, *15*
  blue, 14–17, *15, 16,* 19, 44–45, 47–51, *51*
  blue, filter apps for, 194
  green, 14, 51
  orange, 14
  red, xi, 14–15, *15, 16,* 17, 20–21, 43–45, 50, 52, *53, 90,* 157, 168, 193
  time of day and, 14, *15*
  white, 14, *15,* 17, 18, 21, 44
"light table" experiment, 17
liver, 22, 23

M
Mammoth Cave, 7
melatonin, 15, 16, *16,* 17, 20, 24–25, 34, 36, 39, 45, 49, 50, *51,* 52, 156
metabolism, 22, 33
mice, xxii, 139
misconceptions about baby sleep, 155–58
  "all babies are different," 156
  "imposing a rhythm on baby is unhealthy," 156–57
  "keeping baby awake is unhealthy," 157–58
  "light doesn't matter," 157
  "sleep begets sleep," 26, 95, 156
  "you should never wake a sleeping baby," 95, 96, 158
mood, 3, *5,* 33, 35, 145–48
morning:
  routine for, *92*
  see also waking
Moro reflex, 58

N
naps, 26–28, *30,* 52, *53,* 55, 93–99
  chart on, *191*
  in daycare, 134–35
  determining duration of, 94
  different places for night sleeping and, 60
  feeding and, 83
  last before bedtime, 127
  misconceptions about, 94–95
  newborns and, 82
  nighttime sleep correlated with, 95–97, 118, 124–25, 156
  questionnaire on, 188–89
  reducing, shortening, and dropping, 31, 94–99, 124–28, 157
  resistance to, *30*
  schedules for, 78–83
  skipping, tiredness after, 162
  sleep pressure and, 27–28, *28,* 96, 127
  sleep regressions and, 124–28

sleep training and, 26–28, 94–95, 97

sounds and, 61

spacing of, 98, 127, 157

success story on, 27

trouble going down for, 161

waking a sleeping baby, 95–98

neonatal infant care units (NICUs), 38, 80

newborns, 29, 38–39, 46, 52, 54, 55, 82

feeding of, 80, 83, 86

naps and, 82

schedules for, 73–74, 77–78, *79*, 81

swaddling and, 58–59

white noise and, 61

New York University, xxii

New Zealand Occupational and Environmental Health Research Center, 145

night, 91

feeding at, 19–21, 61, 63, 73, 77, 93, 107

waking during, 39, 56–57

Night Mode, 46–52, *53*, 55, 68–69, 76, 77, 89, *90*, 91, 93, 101, 129

night shift workers, 12, *13*, 35

Nobel Prize, xiii, xviii, 3, 8

nursery school or daycare, 133–34, 157, 161

naps in, 134–35

nursing, 46, 52, 62, 73–74, 83, 84, 160

cell phones and, 50

human pacifier trap and, 83, 86–88

lack of hunger and, 108

nighttime, 77

oxytocin and, 139

schedule for, 78–80

sleep training and, 114

see also food, feeding

O

obsessive-compulsive behaviors, 141–42

opioids, endogenous, 138

oxytocin, xxii, 138–40

P

pacifiers, 61–62

human pacifier trap, 83, 86–88

Pitocin, 139

pituitary gland, 138

plants, 4

postpartum depression, 146–48

postpartum hormones, 139–42

pregnancy hormones, xx, 137–38

prism, *15*

progesterone, 138, 139

prolactin, 139

R

rats, 22–23, 142–43

Rechtschaffen, Allan, 142

red light, xiii, 14–15, *15, 16*, 17, 20–21, 43–45, 50, 52, *53, 90*, 157, 168, 193

Rivkees, Scott, 38

Rockefeller University, xiii, xiv, 3
rocking bassinets, 195
Rosbash, Michael, xiii
Ross, Lori, 147
routines, 39, 59, 74–75, 89–92
    bedtime, 89–91, *90*, 100
    expectations of, 89, 102
    morning, *92*
    see also schedules

S
safe sleep environment, 54–55
St James-Roberts, Ian, 120
St. Joseph's Healthcare Hamilton, 147
schedules, xv–xvi, 39, 55, 73–88,
        127
    adherence to, 100
    bedtime, 33, 38, 76–78
    chart on, *191*
    cluster feeding in the evening,
        85–86
    concerns about imposing, xix,
        156
    crying and, 75, 76, 101
    erratic, *13*
    feeding, 23, 73–76, 78–83, 101,
        156
    for five-month-old, 84–85
    household, 135
    human pacifier trap and, 83,
        86–88
    importance of, xix–xx, 74–76
    for naps, 78–83
    for newborns, 73–74, 77–78, *79*,
        81

questionnaire on, 188–89
repetition and flexibility in,
        100–103
sample, for babies from 0–5
        months, *79*
wake time, 33, 76–78, 160
see also routines
science of sleep, xiii–xix, 1–40
    terminology in, 11–12
    see also circadian clock, circadian
        rhythm
screens, smartphone, computer, and
        tablet, 16, 49, 50–51, *51*, 194
self-soothing, 56–57, 62, 63, 64, 84,
        107, 120, 149
serotonin, *16*, 25, *51*
shift workers, 12, *13*, 35
siblings, 67–69, 161
sickness, xxiv, xxv, 129–32
SIDS (sudden infant death
        syndrome), 54, 62, 63
sleep:
    baby sleep chart, *30*
    circadian clock and, *see* circadian
        clock, circadian rhythm
    conflicting advice on, 155
    development, 94
    disorders, 35
    durations, determining, 94
    environment for, *see* light and
        sleep environment
    erratic, 107–8
    function of, 142–43
    homeostat, 24
    light and, *see* light

logging baby's patterns of, 93–94

misconceptions about, *see* misconceptions about baby sleep

mood and, 145–48

naps, *see* naps

needs for, *see* sleep needs

parental anxieties about, 94

schedules for, *see* schedules

science of, *see* science of sleep

trends in, 101

sleep and nap schedule, 71–103, 156

see also naps; routines; schedules

sleep deprivation, xiii–xiv, 24–25, 33, 35, 96, 142–43, 146–49

brain and, 143–45

rebound sleep and, 25

success story on, 144

sleep increase, 129–32

from sickness, xxv, 129–32

in toddlers, 132

sleeping through the night, xiii–xiv, 105–51

caregivers and, 133–35

chart on, *191*

defined, 118

jagged curve to, 118, *119*

questionnaire on, 189–90

regressions in, 123–28

see also sleep training

sleep needs, 24–27, *28*, 29–31, 68, 93, 94, 101, 124, 125, 127, 156

increased, *see* sleep increase

plateau in, 132

sleep disorders and, 35

sleep pressure, 24–26, *28*, 32, 68, 82, 101

circadian timing and, 37

crankiness and, 85

naps and, 27–28, *28*, 96, 127

sleep problems, xv, xxi, 153–63

common, solutions for, 159–63

in going down at night, 160–61

in going down for nap, 161

tiredness after skipping a nap, 162

tiredness and fussiness when it's not bed or nap time, 161–62

tiredness in evening when bedtime is hours away, 162–63

waking too early, 21, 46–47, 159–60

sleep-related infant deaths, 54

sudden infant death syndrome, 54, 62, 63

sleep sacks, 59, 195

sleep training, xvii, 76, 100, 136

"cry it out" method of, 56, 149

discipline in, xvii, xviii

naps and, 26–28, 94–95, 97

parental brain and, 148–50

self-soothing and, 56–57

signs of readiness for, 107–9, *117*

typical methods for, xiv

weight and, 107, 120

see also Gentle Sleep Training

smartphone, computer, and tablet screens, 16, 49, 50–51, *51*, 194

smartphone apps, 93, 99
  Kulala, 94, 99, 112, 115, 125, 193
social jet lag, 33
Solve Your Child's Sleep Problem
      (Ferber), 56
soothing, 93, 160
  delaying, 63
  in evening, 85
  self-soothing, 56–57, 62, 63, 64,
      84, 107, 120, 149
Stiles, W. S., 19
stress, 138, 141, 147
strollers, 60
sudden infant death syndrome
      (SIDS), 54, 62, 63
sunlight, *15, 16,* 18, *20,* 21, 47, 49, *51,*
      52, 157
suprachiasmatic nucleus (SCN),
      xviii, 9, 10, 12, 14–15, 19, 20,
      22, 35
swaddling, *53,* 58–59, 96
  SwaddleMe blankets, 195
swings, baby, 195

T
television, 16
temperature, 11
testosterone, 138
travel across time zones, 11–12, *13,*
      34–36, 126, 165, 170–86
  in eastern direction, 175, 180
  New York to Beijing example,
      183–85
  New York to Berlin example,
      175–77, *179,* 181–83
  in western direction, 178, 180–81
  see also jet lag

U
University College London, 63, 120
University of California, San
      Francisco, 146
University of Chicago, 142
University of Colorado Boulder, 17
University of Michigan, 100
University of New South Wales, 145
University of Pennsylvania, 143
University of Tokyo, 26–28

V
vacations, 161, 165, 167–69
  see also travel across time zones

W
waking, 38
  morning routine, *92*
  at night, 39, 56–57
  schedule for, 33, 76–78, 160
  siblings and, 68
  too early, 21, 46–47, 159–60
  waking a sleeping baby, 95–98,
      158
Washington University, 58
weekends, 33, 165, 167–69
weight:
  birth, 73–74, 80
  sleep training and, 107, 120
white noise, 61, 68, 194, 195
witching hour, 85–86
Wyszecki, G., 19

Y

Yale University, 38

Young, Michael, xiii, xvii, xviii, 3, 8, 173–75

Young Laboratory of Genetics, xiii

Z

zeitgebers, 10–11, 11, 34–36, 55

   food as, 11, 22–23, 34

   light as, 10, 11, 34

About the Author

Dr. Sofia Axelrod, PhD, is a sleep researcher in the laboratory of Michael W. Young, the winner of the 2017 Nobel Prize in Physiology or Medicine. When she became pregnant with her first child, Dr. Axelrod, a lifelong insomniac, feared she would never sleep again. After the birth of her first baby, she naturally applied her expert knowledge to her baby's sleep. It worked so well that she started spreading the word, working with other families, writing, and talking about the power of sleep science. Through her work, Dr. Axelrod is providing new parents with the thing they need most: a good night's sleep. By educating the public on sleep secrets plucked from the front lines of scientific research, Dr. Axelrod's ultimate goal is to fundamentally improve sleep in our notoriously sleep-deprived society, in particular for parents of young children.

Dr. Axelrod lives with her husband and two young children, Leah and Noah, on the Upper East Side of Manhattan. When she is not investigating the molecular basis of sleep or spending time with her family, she performs classical vocal music on stages in the US and Europe.

Let's Stay in Touch

Working with parents is an integral part of my method, and one that has made my approach so much stronger. This book would not have been possible without you, my sleep-deprived parents, and instead of talking *at* you, I want to keep the dialogue open, because this is a two-way street. I'd love to hear from real parents about their baby sleep experiences, and how my book might have affected them. Please don't hesitate to connect on social media or at how.babies.sleep@gmail.com. To find more information, you can follow me on Twitter (@baby__sleep) or Facebook and Instagram (both @kulalaland), where I post up-to-date articles and information regarding my baby sleep method and research on sleep and circadian rhythms. You can find information about me, my book, and the How Babies Sleep approach at sofiaaxelrod.com.

Kulala
app

Tired of being tired? The Kulala baby sleep app takes all the info from *How Babies Sleep* and puts it at your fingertips. From sleepless nights to resisting naps, enter your child's current sleep problems and get tailored science-based sleep guidance from birth to six years. No more confusion about bed, nap, or feeding times—Kulala creates customized schedules for your baby that automatically update as your child—and family—grows. Whether for a first-time parent or mother of four, Kulala will solve your baby sleep problems and create optimal schedules for the whole family. Learn more at Kulalaland.com/app and use **code HOWBABIESSLEEP** for your complimentary app subscription with the purchase of this book.

GET IT ON Google Play   Download on the App Store

Kulala
lamp

Imagine a night-light that gently helps your baby sleep through the night. Using specially engineered LED lighting, Kulala lamps emit maroon hues that naturally promote baby's sleep hormone for a good night's sleep. Our lamps are designed with real parents in mind and create the perfect sleep environment using a combination of intuitive features. Whether you need to change diapers, feed baby, or simply check on baby, Kulala is right there with you promoting baby's sleep. For older children, Kulala is perfect for reading and as a night-light for children who are afraid of the dark. Kulala lamps feature a beautiful design that fits in every nursery and beyond. Learn more at Kulalaland .com and amazon.com, and use **code HOWBABIESSLEEP** for a special discount with the purchase of this book.

amazon